Advances in Hemodynamic Monitoring

Editor

MICHAEL R. PINSKY

CRITICAL CARE CLINICS

www.criticalcare.theclinics.com

Consulting Editor
RICHARD W. CARLSON

January 2015 • Volume 31 • Number 1

ELSEVIER

1600 John F. Kennedy Boulevard • Suite 1800 • Philadelphia, Pennsylvania, 19103-2899

http://www.theclinics.com

CRITICAL CARE CLINICS Volume 31, Number 1
January 2015 ISSN 0749-0704, ISBN-13: 978-0-323-34172-1

Editor: Patrick Manley
Developmental Editor: Casey Jackson

Critical Care Clinics (ISSN: 0749-0704) is published quarterly by Elsevier Inc., 360 Park Avenue South, New York, NY 10010-1710. Months of issue are January, April, July, and October. Business and Editorial Offices: 1600 John F. Kennedy Blvd., Suite 1800, Philadelphia, PA 19103-2899. Customer Service Office: 6277 Sea Harbor Drive, Orlando, FL 32887-4800. Periodicals postage paid at New York, NY and additional mailing offices. Subscription prices are $210.00 per year for US individuals, $503.00 per year for US institution, $100.00 per year for US students and residents, $255.00 per year for Canadian individuals, $630.00 per year for Canadian institutions, $300.00 per year for international individuals, $630.00 per year for international institutions and $150.00 per year for Canadian and foreign students/residents. To receive student/resident rate, orders must be accompanied by name of affiliated institution, date of term, and the signature of program/residency coordinator on institution letterhead. Orders will be billed at individual rate until proof of status is received. Foreign air speed delivery is included in all Clinics subscription prices. All prices are subject to change without notice. POSTMASTER: Send address changes to Critical Care Clinics, Elsevier Periodicals Customer Service, 11830 Westline Industrial Drive, St. Louis, MO 63146. **Customer Service: 1-800-654-2452 (US). From outside of the US, call 1-314-447-8871. Fax: 1-314-447-8029. E-mail: journalscustomerservice-usa@ elsevier.com (for print support) or journalsonlinesupport-usa@elsevier.com (for online support).**

Reprints. For copies of 100 or more of articles in this publication, please contact the Commercial Reprints Department, Elsevier Inc., 360 Park Avenue South, New York, NY 10010-1710. Tel.: 212-633-3874; Fax: 212-633-3820; E-mail: reprints@elsevier.com.

Critical Care Clinics is also published in Spanish by Editorial Inter-Medica, Junin 917, 1er A, 1113, Buenos Aires, Argentina.

Critical Care Clinics is covered in MEDLINE/PubMed (Index Medicus), EMBASE/Excerpta Medica, Current Concepts/ Clinical Medicine, ISI/BIOMED, and Chemical Abstracts.

Contributors

CONSULTING EDITOR

RICHARD W. CARLSON, MD, PhD
Chairman Emeritus, Director, Medical Intensive Care Unit, Department of Medicine, Maricopa Medical Center; Professor, University of Arizona College of Medicine; Professor, Department of Medicine, Mayo Graduate School of Medicine, Phoenix, Arizona

EDITOR

MICHAEL R. PINSKY, MD, CM, Dr hc, MCCM, FCCP
Professor, Department of Critical Care Medicine, University of Pittsburgh, Pittsburgh, Pennsylvania

AUTHORS

BRENTON ALEXANDER, BS
Medical Student and Research Specialist, Department of Anesthesiology and Perioperative Care, University of California, Irvine, Orange, California

IAN J. BARBASH, MD
Post-doctoral Fellow, Division of Pulmonary, Allergy, and Critical Care Medicine, University of Pittsburgh School of Medicine, Pittsburgh, Pennsylvania

ELIEZER L. BOSE, RN, BSN
PhD Candidate, Department of Acute and Tertiary Care, School of Nursing, University of Pittsburgh, Pittsburgh, Pennsylvania

MAXIME CANNESSON, MD, PhD
Professor, Department of Anesthesiology and Perioperative Care, University of California, Irvine, Orange, California

JOSE CARDENAS-GARCIA, MD
Instructor of Medicine, Division of Pulmonary, Critical Care and Sleep Medicine, Hofstra North Shore LIJ School of Medicine, New Hyde Park, New York

GILLES CLERMONT, MD, CM, MSc
Department of Critical Care Medicine, University of Pittsburgh, Pittsburgh, Pennsylvania

ANDRE L. HOLDER, MD, MSc
Department of Critical Care Medicine, University of Pittsburgh, Pittsburgh, Pennsylvania

MARILYN HRAVNAK, RN, PhD
Department of Acute and Tertiary Care, School of Nursing, University of Pittsburgh, Pittsburgh, Pennsylvania

ALEXANDRE JOOSTEN, MD
University of California, Irvine, Orange, California; Anesthetist, Department of Anesthesiology and Critical Care, Erasme University Hospital, Free University of Brussels, Brussels, Belgium

JEREMY M. KAHN, MD, MS
Division of Pulmonary, Allergy, and Critical Care Medicine; Associate Professor, Department of Critical Care Medicine, University of Pittsburgh School of Medicine; Associate Professor, Department of Health Policy & Management, University of Pittsburgh Graduate School of Public Health, Pittsburgh, Pennsylvania

SHELDON MAGDER, MD
Professor of Medicine and Physiology, Department of Critical Care, Royal Victoria Hospital, McGill University Health Centre, Montreal, Quebec, Canada

PAUL H. MAYO, MD
Professor of Medicine, Division of Pulmonary, Critical Care and Sleep Medicine, Hofstra North Shore LIJ School of Medicine, New Hyde Park, New York

XAVIER MONNET, MD, PhD
Medical Intensive Care Unit, Bicêtre Hospital, Paris-Sud University Hospitals; EA4533, Paris-Sud University, Le Kremlin-Bicêtre, France

MICHAEL R. PINSKY, MD, CM, Dr hc, MCCM, FCCP
Professor, Department of Critical Care Medicine, University of Pittsburgh, Pittsburgh, Pennsylvania

JEAN-LOUIS TEBOUL, MD, PhD
Medical Intensive Care Unit, Bicêtre Hospital, Paris-Sud University Hospitals; EA4533, Paris-Sud University, Le Kremlin-Bicêtre, France

Contents

> Hemodynamic instability as a clinical state represents either a perfusion failure with clinical manifestations of circulatory shock or heart failure or one or more out-of-threshold hemodynamic monitoring values, which may not necessarily be pathologic. Different types of causes of circulatory shock require different types of treatment modalities, making these distinctions important. Diagnostic approaches or therapies based on data derived from hemodynamic monitoring assume that specific patterns of derangements reflect specific disease processes, which respond to appropriate interventions. Hemodynamic monitoring at the bedside improves patient outcomes when used to make treatment decisions at the right time for patients experiencing hemodynamic instability.

> Although use of the classic pulmonary artery catheter has declined, several techniques have emerged to estimate cardiac output. Arterial pressure waveform analysis computes cardiac output from the arterial pressure curve. The method of estimating cardiac output for these devices depends on whether they need to be calibrated by an independent measure of cardiac output. Some newer devices have been developed to estimate cardiac output from an arterial curve obtained noninvasively with photoplethysmography, allowing a noninvasive beat-by-beat estimation of cardiac output. This article describes the different devices that perform pressure waveform analysis.

> Videos of a normal parasternal long-axis view, a normal parasternal short-axis view, a normal apical 4-chamber view, a normal subcostal long-axis view, an inferior vena cava long longitudinal axis view, a severely reduced left ventricular systolic function, a moderately reduced left ventricular systolic function, a hyperdynamic left ventricular systolic function, a right ventricular pressure overload, acute cor pulmonale, a pericardial and pleural effusion,a pericardial tamponade, aortic stenosis, valvular vegetation, papillary muscle rupture, pleural effusion, lung sliding and A lines, lung pulse, lung point, B lines, a consolidation pattern, a noncompressible common femoral vein diagnostic of thrombus, a compressible common femoral vein and artery, a compressible common femoral vein at the level of the saphenous vein intake, a femoral vein at common femoral artery bifurcation, a fully

Critical care ultrasonography is a bedside technique performed by the frontline clinician at the point of care. Point-of-care ultrasonography is conceptually related to physical examination. The intensivist uses visual assessment, auscultation, and palpation on an ongoing basis to monitor the patient. Ultrasonography adds to traditional physical examination by allowing the intensivist to visualize the anatomy and function of the body in real time. Initial, repeated, and goal-directed ultrasonography is an extension of the physical examination that allows the intensivist to establish a diagnosis and monitor the condition of the patient on a regular basis.

Although invasive hemodynamic monitoring requires considerable skill, studies have shown a striking lack of knowledge of the measurements obtained with the pulmonary artery catheter (PAC). This article reviews monitoring using a PAC. Issues addressed include basic physiology that determines cardiac output and blood pressure; methodology in the measurement of data obtained from a PAC; use of the PAC in making a diagnosis and for patient management, with emphasis on a responsive approach to management; and uses of the PAC that are not indications by themselves for placing the catheter, but can provide useful information when a PAC is in place.

Functional hemodynamic monitoring is the assessment of the dynamic interactions of hemodynamic variables in response to a defined perturbation. Recent interest in functional hemodynamic monitoring for the bedside assessment of cardiovascular insufficiency has heightened with the documentation of its accuracy in predicting volume responsiveness using a wide variety of monitoring devices, both invasive and noninvasive, and across multiple patient groups and clinical conditions. However, volume responsiveness, though important, reflects only part of the overall spectrum of functional physiologic variables that can be measured to define the physiologic state and monitor response to therapy.

There is still no "universal" consensus on an optimal endpoint for goal directed therapy (GDT) in the critically ill patient. As in other areas of medicine, this should help providers to focus on a more "individualized approach" rather than a protocolized approach to ensure proper patient care. Hemodynamic optimization needs more than simply blood pressure, heart rate, central venous pressure and urine output monitoring. It is essential to also monitor flow variables (cardiac output/stroke volume) and dynamic parameters of fluid responsiveness whenever available. This article will provide a review of current and trending approaches of the goals of resuscitation in the critically ill patient.

Using What You Get: Dynamic Physiologic Signatures of Critical Illness

Andre L. Holder and Gilles Clermont

The development and resolution of cardiopulmonary instability take time to become clinically apparent, and the treatments provided take time to have an impact. The characterization of dynamic changes in hemodynamic and metabolic variables is implicit in physiologic signatures. When primary variables are collected with high enough frequency to derive new variables, this data hierarchy can be used to develop physiologic signatures. The creation of physiologic signatures requires no new information; additional knowledge is extracted from data that already exist. It is possible to create physiologic signatures for each stage in the process of clinical decompensation and recovery to improve outcomes.

Organizational Approaches to Improving Resuscitation Effectiveness

Ian J. Barbash and Jeremy M. Kahn

Hemodynamic instability and shock are important causes of mortality worldwide. Improving outcomes for these patients through effective resuscitation is a key priority for the health system. This article discusses several organizational approaches to improving resuscitation effectiveness and outlines key areas for future research and development. The discussion is rooted in a conceptual model of effective resuscitation based on three domains: monitoring systems, response teams, and feedback mechanisms. Targeting each of these domains in a unified approach helps clinicians effectively treat deteriorating patients, ultimately improving outcomes for this high-risk patient group.

CRITICAL CARE CLINICS

ISSUE OF RELATED INTEREST

Critical Care Nursing Clinics of North America, September 2014 (Vol. 26, No. 3)
Monitoring Tissue Perfusion and Oxygenation
Shannan K. Hamlin and C. Lee Parmley, *Editors*
Available at: http://www.ccnursing.theclinics.com/

NOW AVAILABLE FOR YOUR iPhone and iPad

Preface

Advances in Hemodynamic Monitoring

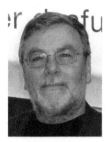

Michael R. Pinsky, MD, CM, Dr hc, MCCM, FCCP
Editor

A fundamental aspect of critical care medicine is the resuscitation and stabilization of patients who present with cardiorespiratory failure due to a myriad of causes. Over the past 50 years since the creation of the subspecialty of critical care medicine, the diseases patients present with, their complexity, our tools to monitor them, and our treatment options have greatly expanded. Central to patient-specific resuscitation and stabilization approaches are the measure and interpretation of their pathophysiologic state, based on physical examination, routine hemodynamic monitoring, specialized tests, and therapeutic challenges.

The worldwide trend of an aging population with greater incidences of comorbidities and immune-compromised states, with regionalization of therapy within the hospital and geographic region, interacts directly with the new and validated monitoring and diagnostic tools. However, within the context of critical care medicine, hemodynamic monitoring implies bedside monitoring. Thus, advanced imaging techniques like NMR and CT scanning are not routinely considered within this context. The newer monitoring modalities and approaches are all addressed in this volume, which was crafted to highlight each.

Thus, for the bedside clinician, this volume addresses this need by presenting the layers of modern hemodynamic monitoring within context. First, we describe the interplay between pathophysiology and bedside measurements, because without a solid understanding of the underlying processes that create the patient's presenting physiologic state, one cannot interpret the resultant physiologic data streams. Monitoring is then divided into the noninvasive and minimally invasive approaches, because if adequate physiologic data can be derived noninvasively, then there is no need for invasive monitoring with all its potential adverse complications. Importantly, the next article is on bedside ultrasound. This tool, long within the domain of cardiology, is now routinely available to all acute care physicians. Potentially, every patient presenting to the intensive care unit with cardiorespiratory insufficiency needs an initial bedside

Crit Care Clin 31 (2015) ix–x
http://dx.doi.org/10.1016/j.ccc.2014.10.001
0749-0704/15/$ – see front matter © 2015 Elsevier Inc. All rights reserved.

echocardiographic examination to define their physiologic state. Presently, this generalized acceptance of the leading role of ultrasound in diagnosis and management of the critically ill patient is embraced more outside of North America than within. However, with the recent Residency Review Committee statement that basic training in ultrasound is an essential aspect of critical care medicine education, this barrier should soon fall. The electronic supplement to this article has an impressive library of ultrasound video images that will serve the reader well in understanding the power of this noninvasive to minimally invasive imaging tool. The volume then continues with invasive monitoring, still the mainstay of hemodynamic monitoring in the most critically ill patients and still extremely important to know its uses and pitfalls. Then, we address the evolving field of "Functional Hemodynamic Monitoring" that uses defined perturbations of the body to note its response to glean knowledge as to the physiologic state. Interestingly, this article would not have been written 20 years ago. Once we understand the pathophysiology, take the appropriate measures, and come to a reasonable conclusion as to the cause of the cardiorespiratory insufficiency, then management is initiated. Within this context, it is very difficult to discuss hemodynamic monitoring outside the context of patient management. Thus, the next article defines the goals of acute resuscitation. From here we take a more systems approach to acute care management by first discussing fused physiologic parameters, smart alarms, and shock indices followed by a discussion on how the organization of the health care system directly impacts the effectiveness of the hemodynamic monitoring approaches described in this volume.

We took the position that each article should be inclusive and complete. Thus, the articles tend to be longer than usual *Critical Care Clinics* articles and fewer per issue. Still, we hope the reader will find this complete overview of monitoring and management useful in their bedside practice. If they do, then our goal has been achieved.

Michael R. Pinsky, MD, CM, Dr hc, MCCM, FCCP
Department of Critical Care Medicine
University of Pittsburgh
606 Scaife Hall
3550 Terrace Street
Pittsburgh, PA 15261, USA

E-mail address:
pinskymr@ccm.upmc.edu

The Interface Between Monitoring and Physiology at the Bedside

Eliezer L. Bose, RN, BSN[a], Marilyn Hravnak, RN, PhD[b],*,
Michael R. Pinsky, MD, CM, Dr hc, MCCM[c]

KEYWORDS

- Hemodynamic instability • Shock • Hemodynamic monitoring

KEY POINTS

- Bedside measures of hemodynamic instability include mean arterial pressure, hypotension, and mixed venous oxygen saturation.
- Causes of circulatory shock can be divided into hypovolemic, cardiogenic, obstructive, and distributive shock, and the hemodynamic patterns are characteristic for each cause.
- The different causes of circulatory shock usually require different types of treatment modalities, making the correct etiologic diagnosis important.
- Pharmacotherapies for hemodynamic instability include vasopressors, inotropes, and vasodilators.
- Technological advances to restore hemodynamic instability include the use of ventricular assist devices and continuous renal replacement therapies.

HEMODYNAMIC INSTABILITY

Hemodynamic instability as a clinical state represents either a perfusion failure with clinical manifestations of circulatory shock or heart failure or 1 or more out-of-threshold hemodynamic monitoring values, which may not necessarily be pathologic. Circulatory shock can be produced by decreases in cardiac output relative to metabolic demands, such as decreased intravascular volume (hypovolemic), impaired ventricular pump function (cardiogenic), or mechanical obstruction to blood flow

Supported in part by National Institutes of Health Grant 1R01NR013912, National Institute of Nursing Research, United States.

[a] Department of Acute and Tertiary Care, School of Nursing, University of Pittsburgh, 336 Victoria Hall, 3500 Victoria Street, Pittsburgh, PA 15261, USA; [b] Department of Acute and Tertiary Care, School of Nursing, University of Pittsburgh, 3500 Victoria Street, 336 Victoria Building, Pittsburgh, PA 15261, USA; [c] Department of Critical Care Medicine, School of Medicine, University of Pittsburgh, 606 Scaife Hall, 3550 Terrace Street, Pittsburgh, PA 15261, USA
* Corresponding author.
E-mail address: mhra@pitt.edu

(obstructive) or by misdistribution of blood flow independent of cardiac output (distributive). The prompt identification and diagnosis of the probable cause of hemodynamic instability, coupled with appropriate resuscitation and (when possible) specific treatments, are the cornerstones of intensive care medicine.[1] Hemodynamic monitoring plays a pivotal role in the diagnosis and management of circulatory shock.

The management of the critically ill patient often requires continual monitoring of hemodynamic variables and the functional hemodynamic status, because of the level of cardiovascular instability that the circulatory shock creates. Patterns of hemodynamic variables often suggest hypovolemic, cardiogenic, obstructive, or distributive shock processes as the primary causes of hemodynamic instability. These different types of causes of circulatory shock usually require different types of treatment modalities, making these differential distinctions important. Diagnostic approaches or therapies based on data derived from hemodynamic monitoring in the critically ill patient assume that specific patterns of derangement reflect specific disease processes, which respond to appropriate interventions.[2]

MEAN ARTERIAL PRESSURE AS A MEASURE OF HEMODYNAMIC INSTABILITY

Organ perfusion is dependent on input organ perfusion pressure and local vasomotor tone. Local vasomotor tone varies inversely with local tissue metabolic demand. For most organs except the kidneys and heart, independent changes in arterial pressure higher than some minimal value are associated with increased vasomotor tone to keep organ perfusion constant and are therefore not entirely dependent on cardiac function and cardiac output. In such situations, cardiac output is important only to allow parallel circuits to maintain flow without inducing hypotension, and cardiac function is important only in sustaining cardiac output and a given output pressure without causing too high a back pressure in the venous circuits. Hypotension, on the other hand, decreases blood flow to all organs. Operationally, mean arterial pressure (MAP) is the input pressure to all organs other than the heart. Diastolic aortic pressure is the input pressure for coronary blood flow. MAP is estimated to be equal to the diastolic pressure plus one-third the pulse pressure between diastole and systole. Over a wide range of MAP values, regional blood flow to the brain and other organs remains remarkably stable because of autoregulation of local vasomotor tone to keep that local blood flow constant despite changing MAP. However, in a previously normotensive patient, once MAP decreases lower than ∼60 mm Hg, then, tissue perfusion may decrease independent of metabolic demand and local autoregulatory processes. As tissue blood flow decreases independent of metabolic demand, then, tissue O_2 extraction increases to keep local O_2 consumption and metabolic activity constant. This process occurs routinely in most individuals and, if transient, is not pathologic. However, if tissue blood flow decreases further than increased O_2 extraction can compensate for, then end-organ ischemic dysfunction follows. Despite the lack of sensitivity of a nonhypotensive MAP to reflect hemodynamic stability, measures of MAP to identify hypotension are essential in the assessment and management of hemodynamically unstable patients, because hypotension must decrease autoregulatory control, and increasing MAP in this setting also increases organ perfusion pressure and organ blood flow.

HYPOTENSION AS A MEASURE OF HEMODYNAMIC INSTABILITY

Hypotension directly reduces organ blood flow, is synonymous with hemodynamic instability, and is a key manifestation in most types of circulatory shock. It also causes coronary hypoperfusion, impairing cardiac function and cardiac output. However, the assumption is often false that because MAP is maintained in low cardiac output shock states by sympathetic tone mediated peripheral vasoconstriction, the patient is not unstable. Intraorgan vascular resistance and venous outflow pressure along with MAP are the 2 other determinants of organ blood flow, and therefore organ perfusion. The normal mechanism allowing autoregulation of blood flow distribution is local changes in organ inflow resistance, such that organs with increased metabolic demand enact arterial dilation to increase their blood flow. If there is hypotension, then, local arterial dilation does not result in increased blood flow, because the lower inflow pressure has minimal effect on the organ perfusion pressure. Thus, hypotension impairs autoregulation of blood flow distribution.[3]

In shock states, normal homeostatic mechanisms functioning through carotid body baroreceptors vary arterial vascular tone to maintain MAP relatively constant, despite varying cardiac output and metabolic demand. Presumably, this vasoconstriction occurs in low cardiac output states to maintain cerebral and myocardial blood flow at the expense of the remainder of the body. In patients with normal renal function, oliguria is the immediate manifestation of this adaptive response, reflecting marked reduction in renal blood flow and solute clearance, despite persisting normal MAP. Normotension does not ensure hemodynamic sufficiency of all organ systems simultaneously. Hence, indirect measures of sympathetic tone, such as heart rate, respiratory rate, peripheral capillary filling, and peripheral cyanosis are more sensitive estimates of increased circulatory stress and hemodynamic instability than is MAP.[4]

Although systemic hypotension can be identified noninvasively using a sphygmomanometer, in the treatment of hypotension not readily responsive to simple maneuvers like recumbency and an initial fluid bolus, invasive arterial catheterization and continuous monitoring of arterial pressure are indicated. There is no consensus as to the absolute indication for invasive arterial pressure monitoring, but caution should be aired in favor of monitoring as opposed to its avoidance in the patient who cannot be rapidly resuscitated. Although peripheral radial arterial catheterization is the most common site for arterial access, femoral arterial catheterization is also available and has the advantage of greater likelihood of successful arterial cannulation in the setting of profound hypotension and shock. The femoral artery is also the preferred site if 1 specific minimally invasive arterial monitoring device (ie, PiCCOplus, PULSION Medical Inc, NJ, USA) use is being considered. However, these issues are addressed in subsequent articles elsewhere in this issue on invasive monitoring and minimally invasive and noninvasive monitoring, respectively. In conditions of marked vasoconstriction associated with profound hypovolemia and hypothermia, central arterial pressure may exceed peripheral arterial pressure because of increased arterial resistance between these 2 sites. Thus, assessing end-organ perfusion parameters like level of consciousness, urine output, and vascular refill are important early measures of the effectiveness of blood flow. Although early attention is appropriately focused on restoring MAP to some minimal threshold level, organ perfusion pressure is MAP minus output pressure. Thus, in the setting of increased intracranial or intraabdominal pressures, cerebral and splanchnic/renal perfusion pressures are less than MAP, respectively, and these compartment pressures need to be directly measured to target an organ perfusion pressure of greater than 60 mm Hg.

MIXED VENOUS OXYGEN SATURATION AS A MEASURE OF HEMODYNAMIC INSTABILITY

One cardinal sign of increased circulatory stress is an increased O_2 extraction ratio, which in the setting of an adequate arterial O_2 content manifests itself as a decreasing mixed venous O_2 saturation (Svo$_2$) in the face of adequate oxygen uptake in the lungs. Svo$_2$ can be sampled only using a pulmonary artery catheter (PAC), whereas central venous (unmixed superior vena cava) O_2 saturation can be assessed using a central venous catheter. The choice of the type of monitoring to be used and how it is interpreted is the subject for the invasive monitoring article elsewhere in this issue. However, low Svo$_2$ values can also occur if arterial O_2 content is low, as is the case with anemia and hypoxemia, or if O_2 consumption is increased, as with muscular exercise.

Muscle activity effectively extracts O_2 from the blood because of the setup of the microcirculatory flow patterns and the large concentration of mitochondria in these tissues. Thus, normal vigorous muscular activity can be associated with a marked decrease in Svo$_2$ despite adequate oxygen uptake and a normal circulatory system and metabolic demand.[2] Muscular activities, such as moving in bed or being turned, fighting the ventilator, and labored breathing spontaneously increase O_2 consumption. In the patient with an intact and functioning cardiopulmonary apparatus, this factor translates into an increase in both oxygen delivery (Do$_2$) and O_2 consumption and a decrease in Svo$_2$ only to the extent that the increased Do$_2$ cannot supply the needed O_2 for this increased demand. Under normal conditions of submaximal exercise, Do$_2$ is the parameter increasing most markedly, although some decrease in Svo$_2$ also occurs. However, in the sedated and mechanically ventilated patient, decreased Svo$_2$ is a sensitive marker of diminished circulation. Although muscle activity is minimal, the diminished flow permits more time for oxygen extraction across the transversed tissue and organ capillary beds. Although there is no level of cardiac output that is normal, there are Do$_2$ thresholds lower than which normal metabolism can no longer occur.[5] Nevertheless, Svo$_2$ can be used as a sensitive but nonspecific marker of circulatory stress, with values less than 70% connoting circulatory stress, values less than 60% identifying significant metabolic limitation, and values less than 50% indicating frank tissue ischemia.[6]

PRINCIPLES OF HEMODYNAMIC MONITORING BASED ON CAUSE OF SHOCK

Weil and Shubin[7] defined circulatory shock in 1968 as a decreased effectiveness of circulatory blood flow to meet the metabolic demands of the body. The heart, vascular integrity, vasomotor tone, and autonomic control all interact to sustain circulatory sufficiency. Circulatory shock reflects a failure of this system and results in an inadequate perfusion of the tissues to meet their metabolic demand, which can lead to cellular dysfunction and death.[8]

Four basic functional causes of circulatory shock can be defined: (1) hypovolemic, caused by inadequate venous return (hemorrhage, dehydration [absolute hypovolemia]); (2) cardiogenic, caused by inadequate ventricular pump function (myocardial infarction, valvulopathy); (3) obstructive, caused by impingement on the central great vessels (pulmonary embolism, tamponade); and (4) distributive, caused by loss of vasoregulatory control (sepsis, anaphylaxis, neurogenic shock, adrenal insufficiency [relative hypovolemia]) (**Table 1**).

Tissue hypoperfusion is common in all forms of shock, with the possible exception of hyperdynamic septic shock, and results in tissue hypoxia and a switch from aerobic to anaerobic metabolism, inducing both hyperlactacidemia and metabolic acidosis. However, hyperlactacidemia is not a reliable marker of ongoing tissue hypoperfusion, because lactate clearance is often delayed or impaired in shock states, and processes such as exercise (seizure activity) and inflammation can induce hyperlactacidemia without cardiovascular insufficiency.[9] Sustained circulatory shock results in cellular damage, not from anaerobic metabolism alone but also from an inability to sustain

Table 1
Categorization of shock states based on the Weil and Shubin nosology

Shock State	Pathophysiology	Disease States	Hemodynamic Monitoring Pattern
Hypovolemic	Decrease in effective circulating blood volume and venous return	1. Primary intravascular volume loss (hemorrhage, capillary leak) 2. Secondary intravascular volume loss (third-space loss, burns, diarrhea, vomiting)	↓ Filling pressures (↓Pra and Ppao) ↓ CO ↑ SVR
Cardiogenic	Primary cardiac failure	1. Impaired contractility (myocardial ischemia/infarction, electrolyte imbalance, hypoxemia, hypothermia, endocrinologic diseases, metabolic poisoning, β-blockers) 2. Pump function (valvulopathy, ventriculoseptal defect, dysrhythmias) 3. Diastolic compliance (LV hypertrophy, fibrosis, infiltrative cardiomyopathies, asymmetric septal hypertrophy, cor pulmonale)	↑ Back pressure to cardiac filling (↑Pra and Ppao) ↓ CO ↑ SVR
Obstructive	Blockage of blood flow in heart's outflow tracts	1. RV outflow obstruction (pulmonary embolism, lung hyperinflation, and pulmonary artery compression) 2. LV outflow obstruction (aortic stenosis, dissecting aortic aneurysm) 3. Cardiac tamponade (pericardial effusion, lung hyperinflation, and atrial compression)	↑ CVP ↓ Ppao relative to CVP ↓ CO ↑ SVR
Distributive	Loss of blood flow regulation	1. Sepsis (increased capillary leak with secondary loss of intravascular volume, and inappropriate clotting in the microcirculation) 2. Neurogenic shock (acute spinal injury above the upper thoracic level, spinal anesthesia, general anesthesia, neurotoxic poisoning, and central nervous system catastrophe) 3. Acute adrenal insufficiency (hyperpyrexia and circulatory collapse)	↓ CVP ↓ Filling pressures (↓Pra and Ppao) ↓ Svo$_2$ ↓ MAP

Abbreviations: ↑, increase; ↓, decrease; CO, cardiac output; CVP, central venous pressure; LV, left ventricle; Ppao, pulmonary artery occlusion pressure; Pra, right atrial pressure; RV, right ventricle; SVR, systemic vascular resistance.

Data from Weil MH, Shubin H. Shock following acute myocardial infarction current understanding of hemodynamic mechanisms. Prog Cardiovasc Dis 1968;11:1–17.

intermediary metabolism and enzyme production necessary to drive normal mitochondrial performance.[10] Metabolic failure caused by sustained tissue hypoxia may explain why surgical preoptimization[11] and early goal-directed therapy[12] improve outcome, whereas aggressive resuscitation after cellular injury has already occurred is not effective at reducing mortality from a variety of insults.[13]

Because most forms of hemodynamic monitoring measure global systemic blood flow parameters like arterial pressure, heart rate, other central vascular pressures, and cardiac output, the assessment of the severity of shock and its initial response to therapy is often limited if monitoring is limited to these global variables alone. Because cellular respiration does not cease when tissue blood flow decreases until some very low level of blood flow occurs, tissue CO_2 production usually continues at a normal rate, resulting in an increased venous PCO_2. Potentially, measuring SvO_2, or alternatively the difference between tissue PCO_2 ($PvCO_2$) and arterial PCO_2 ($PaCO_2$), referred to as the Pv-aCO_2 gap, allows effective tissue blood flow to be assessed, because decreases in capillary blood flow initially cause CO_2 from aerobic metabolism to accumulate.[14] Global measures of circulatory function are being used to determine which of the 4 shock categories is the most likely cause of organ dysfunction, by noting their characteristic patterns or groupings of abnormalities, referred to as hemodynamic profile analysis.[15]

Hypovolemic Shock

Hypovolemia is the cardiovascular state in which the effective circulating blood volume is inadequate to sustain adequate venous return and thus cardiac output to support normal function without invoking supplemental sympathetic tone or postural changes to provide venous return assistance. It is a process of absolute hypovolemia, which can occur through loss of blood, such as with hemorrhage and trauma, or with fluid and electrolyte loss, as with diuresis, diarrhea, vomiting, or evaporation from large burn surfaces, or with severe fluid intake restriction, resulting in dehydration.[16] The normal reflex response to absolute hypovolemia is increased sympathetic tone, causing selective vasoconstriction. Cardiac output is often sustained by this vasoconstrictive maneuver, and venous return is maintained by diverting blood away from the skin, resting muscles, and gut and into the central circulation. The cardinal sign of this circulatory stress is increased heart rate as a result of increased sympathetic tone. If the hypovolemic state progresses, this vasoconstriction becomes inadequate to sustain venous return, and cardiac output decreases. Under these conditions, heart rate increases, but stroke volume decreases more, such that cardiac output declines. With tissue hypoperfusion, increased O_2 extraction occurs across the capillary beds, but eventually even increased extraction fails to sustain aerobic metabolism, and lactic acidosis develops as a marker of tissue anaerobic metabolism.[17] Thus, hypovolemia initiates tachycardia, reduced arterial pulse pressure, and (often) hypertension, with a near normal resting cardiac output, followed by signs of end-organ hypoperfusion (oliguria, confusion) as cardiac output decreases.

Hypovolemic shock represents a decrease in effective circulating blood volume and venous return. It can be caused by primary intravascular volume loss (hemorrhage, capillary leak) or secondary intravascular volume loss (third-space loss, insensible loss through skin with burns, diarrhea, vomiting). The specific findings of hypovolemic shock are decreased cardiac filling pressures (low venous return manifested by low right atrial pressure [Pra] and low left atrial pressure [pulmonary artery occlusion pressure [Ppao]) accompanied by low cardiac output and high systemic vascular resistance (reflexive or sympathetically induced vasoconstriction manifested by high systemic vascular resistance index).[2] Systemic hypotension is the final presentation of hypovolemic shock,[18] and if the clinician waits for hypotension to identify circulatory shock before intervening, ischemic tissue injury is almost always already present.

Cardiogenic Shock

Cardiac pump dysfunction can be caused by left ventricle (LV), right ventricle (RV) failure, or both. LV failure is usually manifested by an increased LV end-diastolic pressure and left atrial pressure, which must exist to sustain an adequate LV stroke volume. Tachycardia is universal in the patient who is not β-blocked. The most common cause of isolated LV failure in the critically ill patient is acute myocardial infarction.[19] However, in postoperative cardiac surgery patients, myocardial stunning can also cause transient LV failure. In acute isolated LV failure, LV stroke work is reduced and heart rate increased. In chronic heart failure, cardiac output may be adequate, or the periphery may have adapted enough to increase O_2 extraction such that tissue hypoperfusion is not present, with the only sign of heart failure being peripheral edema and increased sympathetic tone. However, in acute LV failure, cardiac output may be normal or even increased, as a result of increased sympathetic tone. However, LV filling pressure becomes markedly increased as the increased sympathetic tone decreases unstressed volume, increasing mean systemic pressure and augmenting the pressure gradient for venous return. This situation causes a marked increase in intrathoracic blood volume, which may induce flash hydrostatic pulmonary edema, also known as cardiogenic pulmonary edema. However, neither cardiac output nor systemic vascular resistance is a sensitive marker of LV failure until after cardiogenic shock develops.[20]

The normal adaptive response of the patient to impaired LV contractile function and resulting low organ and tissue perfusion is to increase sympathetic tone, induce tachycardia, activate the renin-angiotensin system, retain sodium by the kidneys, and thus increase the circulating blood volume. In essence, the body does not differentiate its adaptive response to low tissue perfusion caused by either hypovolemic or cardiogenic shock. Fluid retention as a compensatory mechanism, if present, takes time to evolve, whereas acute impairments of LV contractility can occur over seconds in response to myocardial ischemia. Thus, the hemodynamic profile of acute and chronic LV failure can be different. Acute LV failure is manifest by increased sympathetic tone (tachycardia, hypertension), impaired LV function (increased left atrial filling pressure and reduced stroke volume), with minimal RV effects (normal central venous pressure [CVP], unless RV infarction also occurs), and increased oxygen extraction manifested by a low Svo_2. Cardiac output may not be reduced and may be slightly increased early on, as a result of the release of catecholamines as part of the acute stress response.[21] Vascular resistance, therefore, is increased. By contrast, in chronic heart failure, although sympathetic tone is increased, the heart rate is rarely greater than 105 beats/min, whereas filling pressures are increased in both atria, consistent with combined LV failure and fluid retention. Cardiac output is not reduced except in severe chronic heart failure states. A cardinal finding of heart failure is the inability of the heart to increase cardiac output in response to a volume load or metabolic stress state (exercise). Furthermore, because of the increased sympathetic tone, splanchnic and renal blood flows are reduced and can lead to splanchnic or renal ischemia.[22] Although acute heart failure may present with shock, more commonly, patients with preexisting chronic heart failure develop a new illness or acute exacerbation of their heart failure. Thus, their new disease is superimposed on the preexisting heart failure. Such mixed process shock states are often difficult to treat because of the limitations of the patient's cardiac response created by the previous heart failure, and it is easy to induce pulmonary and peripheral edema using routine fluid resuscitation.

Cardiogenic shock represents primary cardiac failure. It can be caused by impaired myocardial contractility (myocardial ischemia/infarction, electrolyte imbalance, hypoxemia, hypothermia, endocrinologic diseases, metabolic poisoning, β-blockers), pump function (valvulopathy, ventriculoseptal defect, dysrhythmias), or diastolic compliance (LV hypertrophy, fibrosis, infiltrative cardiomyopathies, asymmetric septal hypertrophy, cor pulmonale). The specific cardinal findings of cardiogenic shock are increased back pressure to cardiac filling (increased Pra and Ppao) and upstream edema as a result of compensatory fluid retention (peripheral and pulmonary).[2] The hemodynamic profile pattern therefore seen in cardiogenic shock as it progresses is low cardiac output, high Pra and Ppao, and high systemic vascular resistance (reflexive or sympathetically induced vasoconstriction manifested by high systemic vascular resistance index).

Obstructive Shock

Obstructive shock represents a blockage of blood flow in one of the outflow tracts of the heart. It may be caused by RV outflow obstruction (pulmonary embolism, lung hyperinflation, and pulmonary artery compression), LV outflow obstruction (aortic stenosis, dissecting aortic aneurysm), or cardiac tamponade (pericardial effusion, lung hyperinflation, and atrial compression). The specific findings of obstructive shock are often difficult to separate from cardiogenic shock and may be different relative to the ventricle with the obstructive pathophysiology.

The most common cause of obstructive shock is pulmonary embolism and RV outflow obstruction, leading to acute RV failure.[23] However, isolated RV dysfunction can occur in the setting of an acute inferior wall myocardial infarction, and also as a consequence of pulmonary vascular disease (chronic obstructive pulmonary disease, primary pulmonary hypertension) and hyperinflation. Neither pulmonary vascular resistance nor mean pulmonary artery pressure need be grossly increased for RV failure to be present. If pulmonary arterial pressures are greater than 30 to 35 mm Hg, then pulmonary hypertension is probably chronic, because acute increases of pulmonary arterial pressures higher than this level are physiologically tolerable. Increases in CVP of more than 12 mm Hg also reflect fluid retention, suggesting further that RV decompensation or massive volume overload from LV failure has occurred. The most common hemodynamic monitoring pattern in acute pulmonary embolism is that of increased CVP, decreased Ppao relative to the CVP (because preload to the LV is diminished, but LV contractility remains normal), and low cardiac output accompanied by high systemic vascular resistance (reflexive or sympathetically induced vasoconstriction manifested by high systemic vascular resistance index). However, in severe cor pulmonale, RV and LV diastolic pressure equalization occurs, and it is indistinguishable from pericardial tamponade, as acute RV dilation induces tamponade physiology. Echocardiography is useful in making the diagnosis of acute cor pulmonale because it can be performed immediately at the bedside and is noninvasive. Echocardiographic studies show RV diameters greater than LV diameters and a paradoxic intraventricular septal shift. These points are discussed in detail in the article on ultrasonography elsewhere in this issue.

When RV dysfunction predominates and is induced by pulmonary parenchymal disease, it is referred to as cor pulmonale, which is associated with signs of backward failure, increased RV volume and pressures, systemic venous hypertension, and low cardiac output, as well as reduced renal and hepatic blood flow.[24] LV diastolic compliance decreases as the RV dilates as a result of ventricular interdependence, either from intraventricular septal shift or absolute limitation of biventricular volume caused by pericardial restraint. Thus, Ppao is often increased for a specific LV stroke work, giving the erroneous appearance of impaired LV contractility.[25]

Cardiac tamponade, another cause of obstructive shock, can occur from (1) biventricular dilation, limiting biventricular filling caused by pericardial volume limitation; (2) acute pericardial fluid accumulation caused by either effusion fluid (inflammation, severe uremia) or blood (hemorrhage), which needs not be great in quantity; and (3) lung hyperinflation, resulting in mechanical compression of the heart from without, which acts like pericardial tamponade to limit biventricular filling.[26] The first 2 causes are rarely seen, whereas hyperinflation commonly occurs. The cardinal sign of tamponade is diastolic equalization of all intrathoracic vascular pressures (CVP, pulmonary arterial diastolic pressure, and Ppao).[27] Because RV compliance is greater than LV compliance early on in tamponade, there may be selective reduction in RV filling.[28]

Distributive Shock

Loss of blood flow regulation occurs as the end stage of all forms of circulatory shock caused by hypotension but is one of the initial presenting processes seen in sepsis, neurogenic shock, and adrenal insufficiency. The hemodynamic profile of sepsis is one of increased cardiac index, low right and left filling pressures, increased Svo_2, low MAP, and low systemic vascular resistance, consistent with loss of peripheral vasomotor tone and pooling of blood in the vascular system manifesting as a relative hypovolemia.

Sepsis is a systemic process characterized by activation of the intravascular inflammatory mediators, resulting in generalized vascular endothelial injury, but it is not clear that tissue ischemia is an early aspect of this process.[29] Acute septicemia is associated with increased sympathetic activity (tachycardia, diaphoresis) and increased capillary leak, with secondary loss of intravascular volume and inappropriate clotting in the microcirculation. Before fluid resuscitation, this combination of processes resembles simple hypovolemia, with decreased cardiac output, normal to increased peripheral vasomotor tone, and very low Svo_2, reflecting systemic hypoperfusion. LV function is often impaired, but usually in parallel with depression of other organs, and this effect of sepsis is usually masked by the associated hypotension that maintains low LV afterload.[30] Initially, decreased adrenergic responsiveness and impaired diastolic relaxation characterize septic cardiomyopathy. If sepsis remains ongoing, impaired LV contractile function also occurs. However, most patients with such a clinical presentation receive initial volume expansion therapy such that the clinical picture of sepsis reflects a hyperdynamic state rather than hypovolemia, which has been referred to as warm shock in contrast to all other forms of shock.[31]

Neurogenic shock results from an acute spinal injury above the upper thoracic level, spinal anesthesia, general anesthesia, neurotoxic poisoning, and central nervous system catastrophe. All of these states induce a profound loss of sympathetic tone and pooling of blood in the vascular compartment, causing a relative hypovolemic state. In neurogenic shock, the resulting hypotension is often not associated with compensatory tachycardia, and hence, systemic hypotension can be severe and precipitate cerebral vascular insufficiency and myocardial ischemia.[32] Because neurogenic shock reduces sympathetic tone, the biventricular filling pressures, arterial pressure, and cardiac output are all decreased. Treatment consists of reversing the primary process and supporting the circulation with volume loading and an infusion of an α-adrenergic agonist, such as norepinephrine, dopamine, or phenylephrine, to induce vasoconstriction and reverse vascular pooling of blood.[33]

Acute adrenal insufficiency can present with hyperpyrexia and circulatory collapse. This situation is more common than might be realized, based on the epidemiology of adrenal cortical disease, because many patients in the community are receiving chronic corticosteroid therapy for the management of chronic systemic and localized inflammatory states, such as asthma or rheumatoid arthritis. In such cases, the added stress of trauma, surgery, or infection can precipitate secondary adrenal insufficiency, as can the discontinuation of long-term steroid treatment.[34] Patients typically present with nausea and vomiting, diarrhea, confusion, hypotension, and tachycardia. Cardiovascular collapse is similar to that seen in neurogenic shock, except that the vasculature is not so responsive to sympathomimetic support.[35] Because systemic hypotension is a profound stimulus of the adrenocortical axis, measures of random cortisol levels in a patient with systemic hypotension show low values in patients with adrenal insufficiency, and an adrenocorticotropic hormone stimulation test is not needed to make the diagnosis. Accordingly, failure to respond to vasoactive pharmacologic support in a patient who is hypotensive should suggest the diagnosis of adrenal insufficiency, and giving stress doses of corticosteroids usually reverses the unresponsive nature of the shock process.[36] Because there is little detrimental effect of providing adrenal replacement levels of hydrocortisone in the short-term, it is reasonable to start low-dose hydrocortisone (60–80 mg intravenously every 8 hours) while awaiting the response to resuscitation and results of the plasma cortisol test.

CIRCULATORY SUPPORT OF THE PATIENT WITH HEMODYNAMIC INSTABILITY

A summary of the 4 main shock states is provided in **Table 1**. Of the 4 categories of shock, only distributive shock states after intravascular volume resuscitation are associated with an increased cardiac output but decreased vasomotor tone. Thus, cardiac output, stroke work, Do_2, and Svo_2 are decreased in cardiogenic, hypovolemic, and obstructive shock but may be normal or even increased in distributive shock. However, in all conditions, heart rate increases are associated with an increased sympathetic tone (except in neurogenic shock and sympathetic impairment). Hemodynamic monitoring can aid in determining cause of circulatory shock and in assessing response to therapy. Because most forms of circulatory shock reflect inadequate tissue Do_2, a primary goal of resuscitation is to increase Do_2.[37]

If the cause of hypotension is diminished intravascular volume, either absolute or relative, then, cerebral and coronary perfusion pressures must be maintained while fluid resuscitation is begun, otherwise cerebral ischemia and cardiac pump failure may develop and limit the effectiveness of fluid resuscitation.[38] Infusions of vasoactive agents with both α-adrenergic and β_1-adrenergic agonist properties increase both MAP and cardiac output at the expense of the remaining vascular beds, and hence, fluid resuscitation to achieve an adequate intravascular blood volume is an essential cotherapy for sustaining organ perfusion pressure. Isolated vasopressor therapy in the setting of systemic hypotension causes worsening hypoperfusion of the periphery and organs, excluding the heart and brain. Thus, although giving vasopressor therapy in the setting of acute hypotension is often indicated, it is essential to assess volume status as well, because the pathologic ischemic effects of hypovolemia are heightened by isolated vasopressor therapy. Many pathologic states and acute stress conditions are associated with either adrenergic exhaustion or blunted responsiveness to otherwise adequate circulating levels of catecholamines (eg, diabetes, adrenal insufficiency, hypothermia, hypoglycemia, and hypothyroidism). Furthermore, acute sepsis and systemic inflammation are associated with reduced adrenergic responsiveness or relative adrenal insufficiency.[39,40] Thus, even if the patient produces an otherwise adequate sympathetic response, the vasomotor and inotropic response may be inadequate, requiring transient use of potent sympathomimetic agents to sustain hemodynamic stability, and adrenocortical hormone replacement to support relative adrenal insufficiency is also often needed.

PHARMACOTHERAPIES FOR HEMODYNAMIC INSTABILITY

Pharmacotherapies for hemodynamic instability are directed at the pathophysiologic processes that either induce or compound it. Hemodynamic monitoring plays a central role in assessing the effectiveness of these therapies in an iterative fashion. These therapies can be loosely grouped into 1 of 3 processes: (1) those that increase vascular smooth muscle tone (vasopressor therapy), (2) those that increase cardiac contractility (inotropic support), and (3) those that decrease smooth muscle tone (vasodilator therapy).

Infusion of vasopressor agents is indicated to sustain an MAP greater than 60 mm Hg to prevent coronary or cerebral ischemia while other resuscitative measures like volume resuscitation and specific treatments of the underlying condition are initiated. This level of MAP is clearly arbitrary, because some patients maintain adequate coronary and cerebral blood flow at lower MAP levels, whereas others, notably those with either preexistent systemic hypertension or atherosclerotic cerebrovascular disease, may not tolerate MAP decreasing more than 30 mm Hg less than their baseline value.[41] Once an adequate MAP has been achieved and intravascular volume losses corrected, care shifts toward maintaining adequate blood flow to perfuse metabolically active tissues to sustain organ performance and minimizing the detrimental effects of these vasoactive therapies.

Vasopressor Agents for Hemodynamic Instability

Vasopressor therapy can reverse systemic hypotension, but at a price: the only means whereby it can increase systemic MAP is by reducing blood flow through vasoconstriction. Cerebral vascular circuits have no α-adrenergic receptors, and coronary vascular circuits have minimal α-adrenergic receptors, and therefore, their facular beds do not constrict in the presence of exogenous α-adrenergic stimulation. In hypovolemic states vasopressor support may transiently improve both global blood flow and MAP, but at the expense of worsening local nonvital blood flow and hastening tissue ischemia. Initial resuscitative efforts should therefore always include an initial volume expansion component and fluid challenge while diagnostic approaches that identify shock states ensue, before relying on vasopressors alone to support the hemodynamically unstable patient.[42]

Phenylephrine

- Only noncatecholamine sympathomimetic used.
- Differs chemically from other sympathomimetics by absence of a hydroxyl group on position 4 of the benzene ring; this deletion reduces its potency relative to other sympathomimetics.
- Acts as a moderately potent α_1-agonist; used in patients in whom hypotension is caused by decreased arterial elastance (it activates β-adrenoreceptors only at high doses).
- Has a modest direct coronary vasoconstrictor effect, which seems to be offset by autoregulatory mechanisms in the absence of flow-limiting coronary disease.
- Not metabolized by catecholamine O-methyltransferase (COMT), which metabolizes catecholamines; therefore, its absolute half-life is considerably longer than catecholamine sympathomimetics.[43]

- If phenylephrine is used to treat hypotension, it universally causes cardiac output to decrease because α_1-agonist activity results in an MAP increase purely on the basis of the associated increase in vascular resistance and therefore increased LV afterload, but without by β_1 stimulation to assist with improved contractility.
- Its prolonged use is potentially detrimental to tissue blood flow; although its acute use may reverse hypotension and transiently sustain cerebral and coronary blood flow.

Norepinephrine (noradrenaline)

- Has significant activity at α-adrenoreceptors and β_1-adrenoreceptors, resulting in positive vasoconstrictor and inotropic effect.
- Accompanying β_1 activity makes it the α_1-agonist of choice in the patient with hypotension and known LV dysfunction.[44]
- Positive vasopressor effect may enhance renal perfusion and indices of renal function in hemodynamically stable patients; this effect may also be seen at higher doses when norepinephrine is used as a vasopressor in those patients with sepsis.
- If norepinephrine is used to treat hypotension and decreased vasomotor tone, then, outcome is usually MAP increase with minimal changes in cardiac output, because the increase in afterload is balanced by the associated increased contractility.
- However, this balance is also dependent on the LV being responsive to adrenergic stimulation. Maas and colleagues[45] reported that when postoperative cardiac surgery patients had their MAP increased by 20 mm Hg by norepinephrine infusion, cardiac output increased in those with normal cardiac reserve and decreased in those with impaired cardiac reserve. Thus, the cardiac output response to increasing MAP with norepinephrine is variable and dependent on baseline cardiac contractile reserve.

Epinephrine (adrenaline)

- Potent catecholamine sympathomimetic with markedly increased β_2-adrenoreceptor activity compared with its molecular substrate, noradrenaline.
- Has potent chronotropic, inotropic, β_2-vasodilatory, and α_1-vasoconstrictor properties.
- Net vasopressor effect is result of the balance between adrenaline-mediated β_2-adrenoreceptor and α_1-adrenoreceptor stimulation.
- At low doses, this balance may result in no net pressor effect, with a decrease in the diastolic blood pressure. Thus, the effects of epinephrine on hemodynamics are variable and dependent on dosage, perhaps more so than other sympathomimetic agents.
- Like norepinephrine, is known to have potent renovascular and splanchnic vasoconstrictor properties.[38] Clearance rates are variable and mediated by both the COMT and monoamine oxidase systems.

Dopamine

- Most controversial of the clinically used catecholamine sympathomimetics.
- Controversy stems largely from claims for selective, dose-dependent, splanchnic and renovascular vasodilatory properties. Its dopaminergic properties do not reduce the incidence of renal failure in patients with shock when compared with noradrenaline.[46]

- Does stimulate the release of norepinephrine from sympathetic nerve terminals in a dose-dependent manner; this indirect norepinephrine effect accounts for up to half of the clinically observed physiologic activity of dopamine.[47]
- Cardiomyocyte norepinephrine stores are finite, accounting for tachyphylaxis to the positive inotropic effects of dopamine observed after approximately 24 hours in patients with acute myocardial infarction.[48]

Recent clinical trials showing norepinephrine beneficial effects over dopamine

Consensus guidelines and expert recommendations suggest that either norepinephrine or dopamine may be used as a first-choice vasopressor in patients with shock.[49–51] However, observational studies have shown that the administration of dopamine may be associated with mortality that is higher than that associated with the administration of norepinephrine in patients with septic shock.[52–54] The SOAP (Sepsis Occurrence in Acutely Ill Patients) study, which involved 1058 patients with shock, reported that administration of dopamine was an independent risk factor for death in the intensive care unit. In a recent multicenter, randomized, blinded trial comparing dopamine and norepinephrine as the initial vasopressor therapy in the treatment of shock,[55] there was no significant difference in mortality at 28 days between patients who received dopamine and those who received norepinephrine, although dopamine was associated with more severe arrhythmic events than was norepinephrine. Other studies in patients with cardiogenic shock have shown that the mortality was significantly higher in the dopamine group than in the norepinephrine group,[56–58] with higher heart rates in patients who received dopamine as a potential contributor to the occurrence of ischemic events. Clinical trials in critically ill patients at risk for renal failure have also shown no renal vascular saving-effect of low-dose dopamine.[59,60] Recent clinical trials have raised serious concerns about the safety and efficacy of dopamine therapy in the treatment of hypotensive circulatory shock.

Inotropic Agents

Dobutamine

- Synthetic analogue of dopamine.
- Used by continuous infusion as a positive inotrope.
- The improvement in cardiac output noted potentially increases renal blood flow, creatinine clearance, and urine output.
- Also induces vasodilation, which can cause profound hypotension in the hypovolemic patient.
- As a β_1-agonist, increases myocardial oxygen consumption, although autoregulatory increases in coronary blood flow usually fully compensate in the absence of flow-limiting coronary artery disease.
- A noted problem is the development of tachyphylaxis with prolonged (as little as 72 hours) infusions, suggested to be caused by the downregulation of β_1-adrenoreceptors.[61–63]
- A recent randomized, double-blind, placebo-controlled clinical trial in patients with septic shock with low cardiac output and persistent hypoperfusion showed that dobutamine failed to improve sublingual microcirculatory, metabolic, hepatosplanchnic, or peripheral perfusion parameters, despite inducing a significant increase in systemic hemodynamic variables.[64] Thus, changes in measures of macrocirculatory flow may not be translated into changes in microcirculatory tissue blood flow. This potential dissociation between macrocirculatory and microcirculatory is not unique to dobutamine, but may be seen in response to volume resuscitation and both vasopressor and vasodilator therapies.

Dopexamine

- Synthetic dopamine analogue with significant β_2-adrenoreceptor agonist activity.
- Has splanchnic blood flow effects and positive inotropic activity, which have led to enthusiasm for potential usefulness outside its primary indication: decrease of afterload in acute heart failure syndromes with hypertension and oliguria.
- Randomized controlled clinical investigations have reported improvement in morbidity and mortality outcomes when dopexamine was used as the pharmaceutical of choice in achieving goal-oriented oxygen delivery values in perioperative critically ill patients.[65,66]
- Although widely used outside North America, it is not licensed for use in North America.

Phosphodiesterase inhibitors

- Not widely used in management of circulatory shock, but the 2 most commonly used agents in this class are amrinone and milrinone, both bipyridines.
- This class of drugs is also known as inodilators with reference to the 2 predominant dose-dependent modes of action: inotropy and vasodilation.[67]
- Milrinone has shorter half-life and is a more potent (10-fold–15-fold) inotropic agent than amrinone, but otherwise, they are similar agents.[68,69] Both are eliminated by conjugation, with biological half-life of amrinone known to be extended in the presence of congestive heart failure.
- Mechanism of action not precisely known, but at least partially related to inhibition of phosphodiesterase type 3, found in high concentrations in cardiomyocytes and smooth muscle cells; may activate a sodium-dependent calcium channel. Result is increase in intracellular cyclic adenosine monophosphate and calcium, with physiologic effect being improvement in diastolic myocardial function. For this reason, these agents are believed to be positive lusiotropes.[70]
- Clinically used as positive inotropes, given by continuous intravenous infusion after loading dose, with their catecholamine-independent mechanism of action making them theoretically attractive as an inotropic support of choice in patients with potential β_1-adrenoreceptor downregulation.

Levosimendan

- Exerts positive inotropic effects by binding to cardiac troponin C, sensitizing the myofilaments to calcium[71,72] and increasing effects of calcium during systole to improve contraction.
- During diastole, causes calcium concentration to decline, allowing normal or improved diastolic relaxation.[73]
- Also has vasodilatory properties as a result of facilitation of an adenosine triphosphate-dependent potassium channel opening[74] as well as anti-ischemic effects.[75]
- In clinical studies, levosimendan increased cardiac output and decreased cardiac filling pressures and was associated with reduced cardiac symptoms, risk of death, and hospitalization in patients.[76–78]
- Unlike other positive inotropic agents, primary actions of levosimendan are independent of interactions with β-adrenergic receptors.[79] In the LIDO (Levosimendan Infusion vs Dobutamine) study,[73] it was shown to exert superior hemodynamic effects compared with the β-adrenergic agonist dobutamine, and in secondary and post hoc analyses was associated with a lower risk of death after 31 and 180 days.

Vasodilators

Afterload reducing vasodilators act via vascular smooth muscle relaxation. Vascular dilatation is mediated by both nitric oxide (NO)-based and non–NO-based mechanisms, NO being a powerful, locally acting vascular smooth muscle relaxant. Among commonly used vasodilators in hemodynamically unstable patients, both sodium nitroprusside and glyceryl trinitrate (nitroglycerine) function as NO donors. Numerous other non-NO donor vasodilating agents are available, with hydralazine, clonidine, and inhibitors of the renin-angiotensin system being the most commonly used non–NO-based vasodilators in patients with hemodynamic instability. Although uncommonly needed in the management of circulatory shock, their use in combination with vasopressor therapy has recently been advocated to increase microcirculatory flow, because nitrate releasing agents cause microcirculatory flow to increase even in the setting of vasopressor-induced arteriolar vasoconstriction.[80] However, this is an approach still under investigation and not ready yet for general clinical use.[81]

VENTRICULAR ASSIST DEVICES

Ventricular assist devices (VADs) are artificial pumps that take over the function of the damaged ventricle to restore hemodynamic stability and end-organ blood flow. These devices are useful in 2 groups of patients. The first group consists of patients who require ventricular assistance to allow the heart to rest and recover its function. In such situations, it is critical to obtain complete drainage of the ventricle to unload the ventricle, diminish myocardial work, and maximize subendocardial perfusion.[82] The second group consists of patients with myocardial infarction, acute myocarditis, or end-stage heart disease who are not expected to recover to adequate cardiac function and who require mechanical support as a bridge to transplantation.[83,84] Patients on VAD support often require hemodynamic monitoring to assess their cardiovascular state, both in the perioperative state and afterward.

Left Ventricular Assist Device

LV assist devices (LVADs), which are evolving rapidly, are used to treat patients with advanced stages of heart failure. Although the main goals of LVAD therapy are to improve symptoms of heart failure and quality of life, they also reverse pulmonary vascular hypertension in the setting of venous back pressure–induced increased pulmonary vasomotor tone, thus reversing RV dysfunction.[85]

Patient selection is a crucial consideration that determines the outcome of patients who receive an LVAD. In general, patients who receive LVADs have end-stage heart disease without irreversible end-organ failure. For patients who are too ill to undergo heart transplantation, such as those who cannot be weaned from cardiopulmonary bypass, use of a short-term extracorporeal LVAD is a first-line therapy. For patients who are suitable candidates to receive a heart transplant but are unlikely to survive the wait required before transplantation, LVADs are an effective bridge to transplantation.[86]

Complications that could occur in the postimplant period include infection, thromboembolism, and failure of the device. The most common causes of early morbidity and mortality after placement of an LVAD include air embolism, bleeding, right-sided heart failure, and progressive multisystem organ failure.[87] In general, complications are less with the smaller pumps and drivelines and in those that use axial rather than pulsatile flow. Pump thrombosis, a complication with high mortality or one requiring a pump change, can occur, causing an obstruction of the pump,[84,85] but can be treated with tirofiban/tissue plasminogen activator.

Because 60% to 70% of RV systolic power comes from LV contraction,[88] acute cor pulmonale can occur after LVAD insertion. This condition can be corrected by applying therapies aimed at sustaining coronary blood flow (ie, increased MAP) and minimizing any increased pulmonary vasomotor tone (ie, intravenous prostacyclin or inhaled NO). Hemodynamic monitoring often requires echocardiographic support, as described elsewhere in this issue. The unsupported RV is minimally responsive to positive inotropic drug infusion, because most of the beneficial effects of increased inotropy on the RV are derived from increased LV contraction. Thus, volume overload and acute RV dilation are serious concerns and need to be closely monitored using echocardiographic techniques.

Right Ventricular Assist Device

RV dysfunction occurs in clinical scenarios such as RV pressure overload caused by increased pulmonary vascular resistance, cardiomyopathies, arrhythmias, RV ischemia, congenital or valvular heart diseases, and sepsis.[89] The most common cause of increased pulmonary vascular resistance is pulmonary arterial hypertension (PAH), which is defined as the mean pulmonary artery pressure greater than 25 mm Hg with a Ppao, left atrial pressure or LV end-diastolic pressure 15 mm Hg or lower.[90] The critical determinant of patient outcomes in PAH is the functioning of the RV, which has been recognized as an important avenue for further research.[91] Historically, long-term outcomes for patients with PAH are poor. Progressively increasing PAH results in severe RV failure, because the RV, in an attempt to adapt to the pressure overload, becomes hypertrophied and dilated, with diminished systolic and diastolic function. RV failure is the result of PAH and the cause of at least 70% of all deaths from PAH.[92] Mechanical support for the RV may be appropriate in causes in which it is likely to be reversed (ie, acute vasospastic disease) or as a bridge to definitive treatment (ie, lung transplantation). RV assist devices (RVADs) may be used in primary RV dysfunction[93] and have been used with coexisting PAH.[94,95] However, in patients with PAH, there is concern that pulsatile devices may cause pulmonary microcirculatory damage.[96]

Although theoretically an RVAD may be beneficial for decreasing right-side atrial and ventricular filling pressures, decongesting the liver, and increasing LVAD flow, the RVAD itself has complications, with the current RVAD technologies requiring external pumps with a cumbersome drive system, making hospital discharge difficult to achieve.[97,98] Furthermore, it is difficult to assess volume status in patients with RVAD, because the RV is the primary balance between volume and volume response. Thus, no clear guidelines as to minimal CVP values can be made, even when individualized to a given patient's cardiac output, because unstressed intravascular volume can vary widely.

Biventricular Assist Device

The rationale for the use of a biventricular assist device (BiVAD) in patients with heart failure is still controversial. These patients are typically more severely ill preoperatively, have a higher serum creatinine level, and more of them are ventilator dependent before VAD insertion.[98,99] Although the selection of patients for BiVAD support is crucial to obtaining successful outcomes, criteria for predicting the need for a BiVAD have not been well established and remain a major focus for future research. Although rates of survival to discharge have been shown to be similar to LVAD when used after transplantation,[99] patient survival to transplantation is lower with BiVAD than LVAD.[98] Patients on BiVAD therapy are at a greater risk of complications with higher incidences of infection, thromboembolism, and failure of the device caused by twice as many cannulae and pumps.[100] As may be expected, patients with BiVAD are monitored more by their VAD-displayed cardiac output estimates and measures of MAP than central venous O_2 saturation. Volume status and need for vasopressor therapy are usually accomplished through therapeutic trials to observe if changes in cardiac output and MAP occur, rather than on predefined physiologic conditions.

ACUTE KIDNEY INJURY AS A CONSEQUENCE OF CIRCULATORY SHOCK

Fluid resuscitation together with attention to Do_2 are the cornerstones of resuscitation in all critically ill patients.[1] However, acute kidney injury (AKI) is a common complication of circulatory shock and is associated with high mortality.[101,102] Circulating fluid deficits can occur as a result of absolute or relative hypovolemia, resulting in inadequate blood flow to meet the metabolic requirements of the kidneys. Low cardiac output, either as a primary mechanism in cardiogenic shock or a secondary mechanism in the other forms of shock also decreases kidney perfusion. Both of these volume and flow problems must be treated urgently if AKI is to be avoided.[103,104] Although the importance of fluid management is generally recognized, the choice and amount of fluid and fluid status end points are controversial,[28,105,106] requiring special attention to monitoring hemodynamic patterns of fluid resuscitation in patients at risk for AKI.

Risk of Starches to Cause Acute Kidney Injury

Hydroxylethyl starches (HES) are identified by 3 numbers corresponding to concentration, molecular weight, and molar substitution (eg, 6% HES, 130/0.4). According to the number of hydroxyethylations at carbon positions C2, C3, or C6 (degree of substitution), the HES are more or less resistant to degradation by plasma α-amylase. Molar substitution is the most clinically significant number, because it relates to the rate of enzymatic degradation of the starch polymer.[107] Pharmacokinetic characteristics of HES solutions are based on the molecular weight, and degree of substitution and C2/C6 hydroxyethylation ratio.[108] Renal toxicity of HES depends on the level of molar substitution, although a meta-analysis of randomized clinical trials in surgical patients[109] failed to show any difference in the incidence of renal impairment between patients who received low substituted HES and other forms of fluid therapy. However, in intensive care units, renal toxicity has been reported even with low substituted HES, as a result of concurrent sepsis and distributive shock,[110] with the initiation of renal replacement therapies significantly greater in patients who received HES than those who received saline for fluid management.[111]

Continuous Renal Replacement Therapies

In general, critically ill patients receive high daily amounts of volume infusions: continuous infusions, vasopressors, blood, or fresh frozen plasma. Patients with renal failure and in septic shock continue to receive large amounts of fluid resuscitation, thus leading to fluid overload. The consequent positive fluid balance necessitates water removal, with a major consequence of rapid fluid removal being hemodynamic instability.[112]

Daily or every other day conventional hemodialysis (HD) is the standard dialysis regimen for hemodynamically stable patients with renal failure. However, hypotension during HD caused by rapid fluid and solute removal is the most common complication of this therapy and can prolong renal insufficiency in critically ill patients with AKI. The rapid rate of solute removal during HD results in an abrupt decrease in plasma osmolality, which induces further extracellular volume depletion by promoting osmotic water movement into the cells. This reduction in plasma osmolality may contribute to the development of hypotension.

Severe hypotension still accompanies 20% to 30% of HD sessions in patients with AKI.[113] It was for that reason that continuous renal replacement therapy (CRRT) was developed. With CRRT, volume control is more gently continuous and immediately adaptable to changing circumstances (eg, the immediate need for blood or blood products in a patient at risk for acute respiratory distress syndrome). Because of this adaptability, volume overload can be immediately treated or prevented, and volume depletion avoided.

The ideal renal replacement therapy is one that achieves slow yet adjustable fluid removal, to easily meet the highly variable required daily fluid balance. By mimicking urine output, CRRT slowly and continuously removes a patient's plasma water. However, the protection afforded by CRRT is relative and not absolute, because hypotension can still occur if too much fluid is removed or if fluid is removed too quickly, irrespective of the therapy name. Studies comparing CRRT with HD in patients with AKI have not shown a survival benefit for one approach versus the other.[114] It remains a controversial matter as to which clinical parameter (eg, dry weight, MAP, Ppao, Svo_2) or currently available invasive monitoring (eg, central venous catheter, PAC) should be used to define the concept of fluid overload and subsequent therapies to be used for fluid removal.[115]

SUMMARY

Hemodynamic monitoring at the bedside improves patient outcomes when used to make treatment decisions at the right time for patients experiencing hemodynamic instability. For monitoring to provide any benefit, the clinician must be able to use the information to guide management within the context of known physiologic principles and an understanding of the pathologic processes that may be in play. Three basic guiding principles could be used to effectively manage patients with hemodynamic instability associated with signs and symptoms of tissue hypoperfusion. If blood flow to the body increases with fluid resuscitation, then, treatment must include volume expansion. If the patient is also hypotensive and has reduced vasomotor tone, then, vasopressor therapy might be initiated simultaneously. If the patient is neither preload responsive nor showing reduced vasomotor tone and is hypotensive, then the problem is the heart, and both diagnostic and therapeutic actions must be initiated to address these specific problems. Protocolized management, based on existing hemodynamic monitoring technologies at the bedside, is both pluripotential (different monitoring devices can drive the same protocol) and scalable (can alter the resuscitation intensity) and thus lends itself to automation.

REFERENCES

1. Pinsky MR, Payen D. Functional hemodynamic monitoring. Crit Care 2005;9: 566–72.
2. Pinsky MR. Hemodynamic evaluation and monitoring in the ICU. Chest 2007; 132:2020–9.
3. Kellum JA, Pinsky MR. Use of vasopressor agents in critically ill patients. Curr Opin Crit Care 2002;8:236–41.
4. Pinsky MR. Applied cardiovascular physiology. In: Ronco C, Bellomo R, editors. Critical care nephrology. Netherlands: Springer; 1998. p. 1–8.
5. Pinsky M. Functional hemodynamic monitoring: a personal perspective. In: Vincent JL, editor. Yearbook of intensive care and emergency medicine. New York: Springer; 2009. p. 306–10.

6. Rivers EP, Ander DS, Powell D. Central venous oxygen saturation monitoring in the critically ill patient. Curr Opin Crit Care 2001;7:204–11.
7. Weil MH, Shubin H. Shock following acute myocardial infarction. Current understanding of hemodynamic mechanisms. Prog Cardiovasc Dis 1968;11:1–17.
8. Shoemaker WC. Oxygen transport and oxygen metabolism in shock and critical illness: invasive and noninvasive monitoring of circulatory dysfunction and shock. Crit Care Clin 1996;12:939–69.
9. James JH, Luchette FA, McCarter FD, Fischer JE. Lactate is an unreliable indicator of tissue hypoxia in injury or sepsis. Lancet 1999;354:505–8.
10. Crouser ED. Mitochondrial dysfunction in septic shock and multiple organ dysfunction syndrome. Mitochondrion 2004;4:729–41.
11. Kern JW, Shoemaker WC. Meta-analysis of hemodynamic optimization in high-risk patients. Crit Care Med 2002;30:1686–92.
12. Rivers EP, Nguyen HB, Huang DT, et al. Early goal-directed therapy. Crit Care Med 2004;32:314–5.
13. Gruen RL, Jurkovich GJ, McIntyre LK, et al. Patterns of errors contributing to trauma mortality: lessons learned from 2594 deaths. Ann Surg 2006;244:371–9.
14. Silva E, De Backer D, Creteur J, et al. Effects of fluid challenge on gastric mucosal PCO_2 in septic patients. Intensive Care Med 2004;30:423–9.
15. Fiddian-Green RG, Haglund U, Gutierrez G, et al. Goals for the resuscitation of shock. Crit Care Med 1993;21:S25–31.
16. Piper GL, Kaplan LJ. Fluid and electrolyte management for the surgical patient. Surg Clin North Am 2012;92:189–205.
17. Fink M. Does tissue acidosis in sepsis indicate tissue hypoperfusion? Intensive Care Med 1996;22:1144–6.
18. Parks JK, Elliott AC, Gentilello LM, et al. Systemic hypotension is a late marker of shock after trauma: a validation study of advanced trauma life support principles in a large national sample. Am J Surg 2006;192:727–31.
19. Menon V, White H, LeJemtel T, et al. The clinical profile of patients with suspected cardiogenic shock due to predominant left ventricular failure: a report from the SHOCK Trial Registry. J Am Coll Cardiol 2000;36:1071–6.
20. Pinsky MR. Rationale and application of physiologic monitoring. In: Ronco C, Bellomo R, editors. Critical care nephrology. Netherlands: Springer; 1998. p. 33–42.
21. Sapolsky RM, Romero LM, Munck AU. How do glucocorticoids influence stress responses? Integrating permissive, suppressive, stimulatory, and preparative actions 1. Endocr Rev 2000;21:55–89.
22. Gelman S, Mushlin PS. Catecholamine-induced changes in the splanchnic circulation affecting systemic hemodynamics. Anesthesiology 2004;100:434–9.
23. Torbicki A, Perrier A, Konstantinides S, et al. Guidelines on the diagnosis and management of acute pulmonary embolism The Task Force for the Diagnosis and Management of Acute Pulmonary Embolism of the European Society of Cardiology (ESC). Eur Heart J 2008;29:2276–315.
24. Pinsky MR. Heart-lung interactions. Curr Opin Crit Care 2007;13:528–31.
25. Pinsky MR. Clinical significance of pulmonary artery occlusion pressure. In: Pinsky MR, editor. Applied physiology in intensive care medicine. Berlin, Heidelberg: Springer; 2006. p. 53–6.
26. Spodick DH. Pathophysiology of cardiac tamponade. Chest 1998;113:1372–8.
27. Aksoy O, Rodriguez L. Tamponade. In: Askari AT, editor. Cardiovascular hemodynamics. New York: Springer Science + Business Media; 2013. p. 181–96.

28. Pinsky M. Functional hemodynamic monitoring: applied physiology at the bedside. In: Vincent JL, editor. Intensive care medicine. New York: Springer Science + Business Media; 2002. p. 537–52.

29. Hack CE, Zeerleder S. The endothelium in sepsis: source of and a target for inflammation. Crit Care Med 2001;29:S21–7.

30. Pinsky MR, Rico P. Cardiac contractility is not depressed in early canine endotoxic shock. Am J Respir Crit Care Med 2000;161:1087–93.

31. Rabuel C, Mebazaa A. Septic shock: a heart story since the 1960s. Intensive Care Med 2006;32:799–807.

32. Kiss ZH, Tator CH. Neurogenic shock. In: Geller ER, editor. Shock and resuscitation. New York: McGraw-Hill; 1993. p. 421–40.

33. Müllner M, Urbanek B, Havel C, et al. Vasopressors for shock. Cochrane Database Syst Rev 2004;(3):CD003709.

34. Sabharwal P, Fishel RS, Breslow MJ. Adrenal insufficiency–an unusual cause of shock in postoperative patients. Endocr Pract 1998;4:387–90.

35. Bouachour G, Tirot P, Varache N, et al. Hemodynamic changes in acute adrenal insufficiency. Intensive Care Med 1994;20:138–41.

36. Claussen MS, Landercasper J, Cogbill TH. Acute adrenal insufficiency presenting as shock after trauma and surgery: three cases and review of the literature. J Trauma 1992;32:94–100.

37. Moore FA, McKinley BA, Moore EE. The next generation in shock resuscitation. Lancet 2004;363:1988–96.

38. Mehta NK, Pinsky MR. Pharmacologic support of the hemodynamically unstable patient. In: Ronco C, Bellomo R, editors. Critical care nephrology. Netherlands: Springer; 1998. p. 43–50.

39. Hennein HA, Ebba H, Rodriguez JL, et al. Relationship of the proinflammatory cytokines to myocardial ischemia and dysfunction after uncomplicated coronary revascularization. J Thorac Cardiovasc Surg 1994;108:626–35.

40. Oddis CV, Finkel MS. Cytokines and nitric oxide synthase inhibitor as mediators of adrenergic refractoriness in cardiac myocytes. Eur J Pharmacol 1997;320:167–74.

41. Pinsky M. Protocolized cardiovascular management based on ventricular-arterial coupling. In: Pinsky M, Payen D, editors. Functional hemodynamic monitoring. Berlin, Heidelberg: Springer; 2005. p. 381–95.

42. Pinsky MR. Assessment of indices of preload and volume responsiveness. Curr Opin Crit Care 2005;11:235–9.

43. Westfall TC, Westfall DP. Adrenergic agonists and antagonists. In: Brunton LL, Lazo JS, Parker KL, editors. Goodman and Gilman's the pharmacological basis of therapeutics. 11th edition. New York: McGraw-Hill; 2006. p. 237–315.

44. Skomedal T, Borthne K, Aass H, et al. Comparison between alpha-1 adrenoceptor-mediated and beta adrenoceptor-mediated inotropic components elicited by norepinephrine in failing human ventricular muscle. J Pharmacol Exp Ther 1997;280:721–9.

45. Maas JJ, Pinsky MR, de Wilde RB, et al. Cardiac output response to norepinephrine in postoperative cardiac surgery patients: interpretation with venous return and cardiac function curves. Crit Care Med 2013;41:143–50.

46. Perdue PW, Balser JR, Lipsett PA, et al. "Renal dose" dopamine in surgical patients: dogma or science? Ann Surg 1998;227:470.

47. Smith A. Mechanisms involved in the release of noradrenaline from sympathetic nerves. Br Med Bull 1973;29:123–9.

48. Parissis JT, Farmakis D, Nieminen M. Classical inotropes and new cardiac enhancers. Heart Fail Rev 2007;12:149–56.
49. Hollenberg SM, Ahrens TS, Annane D, et al. Practice parameters for hemodynamic support of sepsis in adult patients: 2004 update. Crit Care Med 2004; 32:1928–48.
50. Antman EM, Anbe DT, Armstrong PW, et al. ACC/AHA guidelines for the management of patients with ST-elevation myocardial infarction–executive summary. A report of the American College of Cardiology/American Heart Association Task Force on Practice Guidelines. J Am Coll Cardiol 2004;44:671–719.
51. Dellinger RP, Levy MM, Carlet JM, et al. Surviving Sepsis Campaign: international guidelines for management of severe sepsis and septic shock: 2008. Intensive Care Med 2008;34:17–60.
52. Sakr Y, Reinhart K, Vincent JL, et al. Does dopamine administration in shock influence outcome? Results of the Sepsis Occurrence in Acutely Ill Patients (SOAP) Study. Crit Care Med 2006;34:589–97.
53. Martin C, Viviand X, Leone M, et al. Effect of norepinephrine on the outcome of septic shock. Crit Care Med 2000;28:2758–65.
54. Boulain T, Runge I, Bercault N, et al. Dopamine therapy in septic shock: detrimental effect on survival? J Crit Care 2009;24:575–82.
55. De Backer D, Biston P, Devriendt J, et al. Comparison of dopamine and norepinephrine in the treatment of shock. N Engl J Med 2010;362:779–89.
56. Loeb HS, Winslow EB, Rahimtoola SH, et al. Acute hemodynamic effects of dopamine in patients with shock. Circulation 1971;44:163–73.
57. Winslow EJ, Loeb HS, Rahimtoola SH, et al. Hemodynamic studies and results of therapy in 50 patients with bacteremic shock. Am J Med 1973;54: 421–32.
58. Ungar A, Fumagalli S, Marini M, et al. Renal, but not systemic, hemodynamic effects of dopamine are influenced by the severity of congestive heart failure. Crit Care Med 2004;32:1125–9.
59. Bellomo R, Chapman M, Finfer S, et al. Low-dose dopamine in patients with early renal dysfunction: a placebo-controlled randomised trial. Australian and New Zealand Intensive Care Society (ANZICS) Clinical Trials Group. Lancet 2000;356:2139–43.
60. Jones D, Bellomo R. Renal-dose dopamine: from hypothesis to paradigm to dogma to myth and, finally, superstition? J Intensive Care Med 2005;20: 199–211.
61. Klein NA, Siskind SJ, Frishman WH, et al. Hemodynamic comparison of intravenous amrinone and dobutamine in patients with chronic congestive heart failure. Am J Cardiol 1981;48:170–5.
62. Unverferth DV, Blanford M, Kates RE, et al. Tolerance to dobutamine after a 72 hour continuous infusion. Am J Med 1980;69:262–6.
63. O'Connor CM, Gattis WA, Uretsky BF, et al. Continuous intravenous dobutamine is associated with an increased risk of death in patients with advanced heart failure: insights from the Flolan International Randomized Survival Trial (FIRST). Am Heart J 1999;138:78–86.
64. Hernandez G, Bruhn A, Luengo C, et al. Effects of dobutamine on systemic, regional and microcirculatory perfusion parameters in septic shock: a randomized, placebo-controlled, double-blind, crossover study. Intensive Care Med 2013;39:1435–43.
65. Hayes MA, Timmins AC, Yau E, et al. Elevation of systemic oxygen delivery in the treatment of critically ill patients. N Engl J Med 1994;330:1717–22.

66. Boyd O, Grounds RM, Bennett ED. A randomized clinical trial of the effect of deliberate perioperative increase of oxygen delivery on mortality in high-risk surgical patients. JAMA 1993;270:2699–707.
67. Dei Cas L, Metra M, Visioli O. Clinical pharmacology of inodilators. J Cardiovasc Pharmacol 1989;14:S60–71.
68. Alousi A, Johnson D. Pharmacology of the bipyridines: amrinone and milrinone. Circulation 1986;73:III10–24.
69. Earl C, Linden J, Weglicki W. Biochemical mechanisms for the inotropic effect of the cardiotonic drug milrinone. J Cardiovasc Pharmacol 1985;8:864–72.
70. Lipskaia L, Chemaly ER, Hadri L, et al. Sarcoplasmic reticulum Ca^{2+} ATPase as a therapeutic target for heart failure. Expert Opin Biol Ther 2010;10:29–41.
71. Haikala H, Kaivola J, Nissinen E, et al. Cardiac troponin C as a target protein for a novel calcium sensitizing drug, levosimendan. J Mol Cell Cardiol 1995;27:1859–66.
72. Haikala H, Nissinen E, Etemadzadeh E, et al. Troponin C-mediated calcium sensitization induced by levosimendan does not impair relaxation. J Cardiovasc Pharmacol 1995;25:794–801.
73. Follath F, Cleland J, Just H, et al. Efficacy and safety of intravenous levosimendan compared with dobutamine in severe low-output heart failure (the LIDO study): a randomised double-blind trial. Lancet 2002;360:196–202.
74. Yokoshiki H, Katsube Y, Sunagawa M, et al. Levosimendan, a novel Ca^{+2} sensitizer, activates the glibenclamide-sensitive K^+ channel in rat arterial myocytes. Eur J Pharmacol 1997;333:249–59.
75. Kersten JR, Montgomery MW, Pagel PS, et al. Levosimendan, a new positive inotropic drug, decreases myocardial infarct size via activation of KATP channels. Anesth Analg 2000;90:5.
76. Nieminen MS, Akkila J, Hasenfuss G, et al. Hemodynamic and neurohumoral effects of continuous infusion of levosimendan in patients with congestive heart failure. J Am Coll Cardiol 2000;36:1903–12.
77. Slawsky MT, Colucci WS, Gottlieb SS, et al. Acute hemodynamic and clinical effects of levosimendan in patients with severe heart failure. Circulation 2000;102:2222–7.
78. Moiseyev V, Poder P, Andrejevs N, et al. Safety and efficacy of a novel calcium sensitizer, levosimendan, in patients with left ventricular failure due to an acute myocardial infarction. A randomized, placebo-controlled, double-blind study (RUSSLAN). Eur Heart J 2002;23:1422–32.
79. Haikala H, Kaheinen P, Levijoki J, et al. The role of cAMP-and cGMP-dependent protein kinases in the cardiac actions of the new calcium sensitizer, levosimendan. Cardiovasc Res 1997;34:536–46.
80. Trzeciak S, McCoy JV, Dellinger RP, et al. Early increases in microcirculatory perfusion during protocol-directed resuscitation are associated with reduced multi-organ failure at 24 h in patients with sepsis. Intensive Care Med 2008;34:2210–7.
81. De Backer D, Hollenberg S, Boerma C, et al. How to evaluate the microcirculation: report of a round table conference. Crit Care 2007;11(5):R101.
82. Emery RW, Joyce LD. Directions in cardiac assistance. J Card Surg 1991;6:400–14.
83. Pae W, Pierce W. Temporary left ventricular assistance in acute myocardial infarction and cardiogenic shock: rationale and criteria for utilization. Chest 1981;79:692–5.
84. Frazier O, Rose EA, Macmanus Q, et al. Multicenter clinical evaluation of the Heart-Mate 1000 IP left ventricular assist device. Ann Thorac Surg 1992;53:1080–90.

85. Lund LH, Matthews J, Aaronson K. Patient selection for left ventricular assist devices. Eur J Heart Fail 2010;12:434–43.
86. Goldstein DJ, Oz MC, Rose EA. Implantable left ventricular assist devices. N Engl J Med 1998;339:1522–33.
87. Potapov EV, Stepanenko A, Krabatsch T, et al. Managing long-term complications of left ventricular assist device therapy. Curr Opin Cardiol 2011;26:237–44.
88. Damiano R, La Follette P, Cox J, et al. Significant left ventricular contribution to right ventricular systolic function. Am J Physiol 1991;261:H1514–24.
89. Simon MA, Pinsky MR. Right ventricular dysfunction and failure in chronic pressure overload. Cardiol Res Pract 2011;23:5680–95.
90. McLaughlin VV, Archer SL, Badesch DB, et al. ACCF/AHA 2009 Expert Consensus document on pulmonary hypertension. J Am Coll Cardiol 2009;53:1573–619.
91. Voelkel NF, Quaife RA, Leinwand LA, et al. Right ventricular function and failure report of a National Heart, Lung, and Blood Institute Working Group on cellular and molecular mechanisms of right heart failure. Circulation 2006;114:1883–91.
92. D'Alonzo GE, Barst RJ, Ayres SM, et al. Survival in patients with primary pulmonary hypertension–results from a national prospective registry. Ann Intern Med 1991;115:343–9.
93. Giesler GM, Gomez JS, Letsou G, et al. Initial report of percutaneous right ventricular assist for right ventricular shock secondary to right ventricular infarction. Catheter Cardiovasc Interv 2006;68:263–6.
94. Fonger J, Borkon A, Baumgartner W, et al. Acute right ventricular failure following heart transplantation: improvement with prostaglandin E1 and right ventricular assist. J Heart transplant 1985;5:317–21.
95. Nagarsheth NP, Pinney S, Bassily-Marcus A, et al. Successful placement of a right ventricular assist device for treatment of a presumed amniotic fluid embolism. Anesth Analg 2008;107:962–4.
96. Berman M, Tsui S, Vuylsteke A, et al. Life-threatening right ventricular failure in pulmonary hypertension: RVAD or ECMO? J Heart Lung Transplant 2008;27:1188–9.
97. Chen JM, Levin HR, Rose EA, et al. Experience with right ventricular assist devices for perioperative right-sided circulatory failure. Ann Thorac Surg 1996;61:305–10.
98. Farrar DJ, Hill JD, Pennington DG, et al. Preoperative and postoperative comparison of patients with univentricular and biventricular support with the Thoratec ventricular assist device as a bridge to cardiac transplantation. J Thorac Cardiovasc Surg 1997;113:202–9.
99. Tsukui H, Teuteberg JJ, Murali S, et al. Biventricular assist device utilization for patients with morbid congestive heart failure: a justifiable strategy. Circulation 2005;112:I65–72.
100. Pennington D, Reedy J, Swartz M, et al. Univentricular versus biventricular assist device support. J Heart Lung Transplant 1990;10:258–63.
101. Chertow M, Glenn M, Levy M, et al. Independent association between acute renal failure and mortality following cardiac surgery. Am J Med 1998;104:343–8.
102. Bellomo R, Kellum J, Ronco C. Acute renal failure: time for consensus. Intensive Care Med 2001;27:1685–8.
103. Blow O, Magliore L, Claridge JA, et al. The golden hour and the silver day: detection and correction of occult hypoperfusion within 24 hours improves outcome from major trauma. J Trauma 1999;47:964.

104. Claridge JA, Crabtree TD, Pelletier SJ, et al. Persistent occult hypoperfusion is associated with a significant increase in infection rate and mortality in major trauma patients. J Trauma 2000;48:8.
105. Michard F, Boyssats S, Chemla D, et al. Relation between respiratory changes in arterial pulse pressure and fluid responsiveness in septic patients with acute circulatory failure. Am J Respir Crit Care Med 2000;162:134–8.
106. Pinsky MR. Pulmonary artery occlusion pressure. In: Pinsky M, Brochard L, Hedenstierna G, et al, editors. Applied physiology in intensive care medicine 1. Berlin, Heidelberg: Springer; 2012. p. 83–6.
107. Westphal M, James MF, Kozek-Langenecker S, et al. Hydroxyethyl starches: different products–different effects. Anesthesiology 2009;111:187–202.
108. Ragaller MJ, Theilen H, Koch T. Volume replacement in critically ill patients with acute renal failure. J Am Soc Nephrol 2001;12:S33–9.
109. Van Der Linden P, James M, Mythen M, et al. Safety of modern starches used during surgery. Anesth Analg 2013;116:35–48.
110. Sear JW. Kidney dysfunction in the postoperative period. Br J Anaesth 2005;95: 20–32.
111. Rahbari NN, Zimmermann JB, Schmidt T, et al. Meta-analysis of standard, restrictive and supplemental fluid administration in colorectal surgery. Br J Surg 2009;96:331–41.
112. Ronco C, Bellomo R, Ricci Z. Continuous renal replacement therapy in critically ill patients. Nephrol Dial Transplant 2001;16(suppl 5):67–72.
113. Hakim RM, Wingard RL, Parker RA. Effect of the dialysis membrane in the treatment of patients with acute renal failure. N Engl J Med 1994;331:1338–42.
114. Jun M, Heerspink HJL, Ninomiya T, et al. Intensities of renal replacement therapy in acute kidney injury: a systematic review and meta-analysis. Clin J Am Soc Nephrol 2010;5:956–63.
115. Vincent JL, Abraham E, Kochanek P, et al. Textbook of critical care: expert consult premium. Philadelphia: Elsevier Health Sciences; 2011.

Minimally Invasive Monitoring

Xavier Monnet, MD, PhD[a,b],*, Jean-Louis Teboul, MD, PhD[a,b]

KEYWORDS

- Hemodynamic monitoring • Cardiac output • Arterial pressure
- Pulse contour analysis • Vascular resistance • Thermodilution

KEY POINTS

- The main advantage of pulse contour analysis is to provide a continuous real-time estimation of cardiac output.
- Calibrated pulse contour analysis devices provide a reliable estimation of cardiac output but are invasive and require frequent recalibrations.
- The reliability of devices using uncalibrated pulse contour analysis is low when vascular resistance changes to a large extent. These devices are more suitable for the perioperative setting than for intensive care units.
- Pulse contour analysis of noninvasive tracings of arterial pressure still needs to be improved.

INTRODUCTION

For many years, the measurement of cardiac output in operating rooms and intensive care units could be performed only with the pulmonary artery catheter. The popularity of the pulmonary artery catheter has progressively declined and some alternative techniques have been developed during recent years,[1] mainly because catheters are invasive, cumbersome to set up, and some of the variables it provides can be difficult to measure and interpret appropriately. Among the alternative techniques, arterial pressure waveform analysis infers cardiac output from the systemic arterial pressure curve. Some of these arterial pressure waveform analysis devices only need an arterial catheter for this purpose and can be considered as minimally invasive. Pulse contour analysis was recently developed for arterial curves that are recorded in a noninvasive way.

Conflicts of interest: Professors X. Monnet and J-L. Teboul are members of the medical advisory board of Pulsion Medical Systems.

[a] Medical Intensive Care Unit, Bicêtre Hospital, Paris-Sud University Hospitals, 78, rue du Général Leclerc, F-94270 Le Kremlin-Bicêtre, France; [b] EA4533, Paris-Sud University, 63 rue Gabriel Péri, F-94270 Le Kremlin-Bicêtre, France
* Corresponding author. Service de réanimation médicale, Hôpital de Bicêtre, 78 rue du Général Leclerc, 94 270 Le Kremlin-Bicêtre, France.
E-mail address: xavier.monnet@bct.aphp.fr

Crit Care Clin 31 (2015) 25–42
http://dx.doi.org/10.1016/j.ccc.2014.08.002
0749-0704/15/$ – see front matter © 2015 Elsevier Inc. All rights reserved.
criticalcare.theclinics.com

This article first summarizes the technological principles of pulse contour analysis. In particular, it explains how devices differ in whether or not they need to be calibrated. The literature on the reliability of arterial pressure waveform analysis for estimating cardiac output is reviewed. In addition, the role of such devices with respect to the other hemodynamic monitoring devices is discussed.

PRINCIPLES OF ARTERIAL PRESSURE WAVEFORM ANALYSIS

Two types of device that use arterial pressure waveform analysis have been developed. Some of them (PiCCO by Pulsion Medical Systems, Munich, Germany; LiDCOplus by LiDCO, London, United Kingdom; and VolumeView/EV1000 by Edwards Lifesciences, Irvine, CA) calibrate the pressure waveform analysis with an independent measurement of cardiac output done by transpulmonary dilution. Some other devices (FloTrac/Vigileo by Edwards Lifesciences; LiDCOrapid by LiDCO; Most-Care by Vytech Health, Padova, Italy; and ProAQT/Pulsioflex by Pulsion Medical Systems) do not require any calibration for pressure waveform analysis and are minimally invasive because they only require a standard arterial catheter.

This article briefly describes the functioning principle of both kinds of pressure waveform analysis device. However, the precise algorithms used by the devices are not disclosed by the manufacturers.

Calibrated Devices

These devices integrate 2 independent techniques for measuring cardiac output: arterial pressure waveform analysis and transpulmonary dilution (with cold saline for PiCCO and VolumeView/EV1000, and with lithium for LiDCOplus).

PiCCO and VolumeView/EV1000

Principles common to both devices The PiCCO and VolumeView/EV1000 devices use a pressure waveform analysis that is based on the principle that stroke volume is proportional to arterial pulse pressure and inversely proportional to arterial compliance. In the early 1990s, Wesseling and colleagues[2] computed the aortic flow from the systemic arterial pressure in humans. They simulated a 3-element model including the characteristic impedance of the aorta, the arterial compliance, and systemic vascular resistance (**Fig. 1**). They described for the first time that it is possible to monitor cardiac output continuously from pulse contour analysis.[2]

Based on this principle, all devices estimating cardiac output from pressure waveform analysis record the arterial pressure curve from a peripheral artery and automatically compute cardiac output from it. Overall, for most devices, the analysis is supported by 4 principles:

1. The amplitude of the pressure curve of the aorta is proportional to stroke volume and to a multiplication factor k.
2. k is inversely proportional to the arterial compliance.
3. The arterial pressure at the periphery is different from the arterial pressure at the aortic level (see **Fig. 1**). This difference is called the pulse wave amplification phenomenon. Because of the reduction of arterial diameter from the aorta to the periphery, the amplitude of the arterial pressure signal increases along the arterial tree.
4. The amplification of pulse along the arterial tree depends on the arterial resistance.

As a result, arterial pressure waveform analysis devices must:

1. Analyze the geometry of the arterial pressure curve signal
2. Estimate the arterial compliance

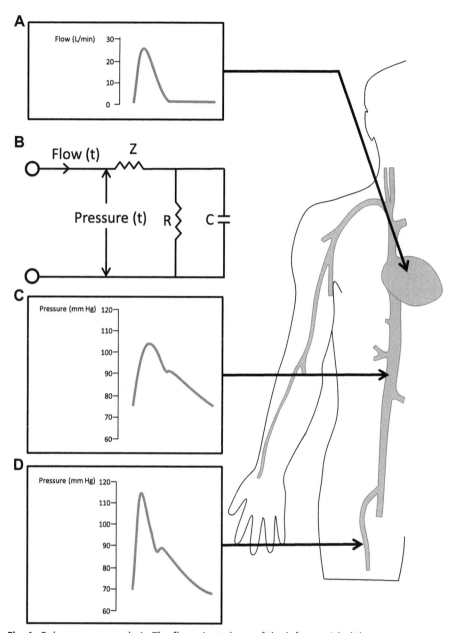

Fig. 1. Pulse pressure analysis. The flow ejected out of the left ventricle (*A*) generates a pressure at the aortic level (*C*) and at the femoral level (*D*). The relationship between flow and the aortic pressure can be represented in a 3-element model (*B*), according to Wesseling.[2] In this model, Z is the characteristic impedance of the aorta, t is time, R is the total arterial resistance, and C is the total compliance of the arterial system.

3. Estimate the aortic pressure from a peripheral arterial pressure
4. Take into account the level of arterial tone

PiCCO With this device, pulse contour analysis estimates cardiac output by integrating the area under the systolic part of the arterial curve and dividing it by the aortic compliance.[3] In addition to the area under the systolic part of the curve, the system takes into account some geometric properties of the pressure curve, such as the time of the dicrotic notch. The arterial compliance is estimated by a proprietary algorithm when calibration is performed (ie, at each time cardiac output is measured by transpulmonary thermodilution). In addition, the algorithm takes into account the systemic vascular resistance, which is continuously tracked by another proprietary algorithm.

Resistance is estimated by dividing mean arterial pressure by the value of cardiac output obtained by transpulmonary thermodilution.

Calibrating the PiCCO pulse contour analysis by transpulmonary thermodilution is justified because the latter technique provides an estimation of cardiac output that is reliable[4] and precise[5] compared with classic pulmonary thermodilution. Moreover, transpulmonary thermodilution has the advantage of providing many other variables besides cardiac output, such as extravascular lung water,[6] pulmonary vascular permeability, the cardiac function index (a marker of the cardiac systolic function),[7] and the global end-diastolic volume (a marker of cardiac preload).[4] All these additional variables may be helpful in the decision-making process of hemodynamic resuscitation.

Between 2 calibrations, compliance and resistance are constantly reassessed by an algorithm that mainly takes into account the arterial pressure curve and the first derivative of pressure on time according to the equation:

$$SV = Cal \times \int systole\ [P(t)/SVR + C(p) \times dp/dt] \times dt$$

where *SV* is stroke volume; *Cal* is calibrating factor; *P(t)* is arterial pressure; *SVR* is systemic vascular resistance; and *C(p)* is arterial compliance, which is calculated from arterial pressure.

With this constant reassessment of the arterial compliance, the system tends to adapt its estimation of cardiac output to the modifications of the hemodynamic status between 2 calibrations by transpulmonary thermodilution.

Because it requires transpulmonary thermodilution and because transpulmonary thermodilution requires a central venous catheter and a large-diameter femoral arterial catheter, the PiCCO device must be considered more as less invasive than as minimally invasive.[8]

Another disadvantage of the PiCCO device is that it requires frequent recalibrations. A study found that the estimation of cardiac output by pulse contour analysis became insufficiently reliable if the previous calibration was performed more than 1 hour before.[9] The drift of pulse contour analysis–derived cardiac output is particularly important if arterial resistance changes to a large extent. In practice, this does not mean that the pulse contour analysis should be systematically recalibrated every hour in every patient, but rather that, in case of hemodynamic instability, calibration should be performed if it has not been performed for more than 1 hour.

Volumeview/EV1000 The VolumeView/EV1000 device is another transpulmonary thermodilution device that, in many aspects, works like the PiCCO, at least as far as can be ascertained from the manufacturer. Like the PiCCO, the system uses transpulmonary thermodilution to calibrate the pulse contour analysis–derived estimation of cardiac output. The estimation of cardiac output is based on the algorithm that is also used by the FloTrac/Vigileo device (discussed later). As with the PiCCO device, because of the arterial catheter required by transpulmonary thermodilution, the VolumeView/EV1000 is less invasive rather than minimally invasive.

LiDCOplus

The LiDCOplus calibrates pressure waveform analysis by lithium transpulmonary dilution. With this technique, lithium chloride is injected as an intravenous bolus into a central vein, and its concentration in arterial blood is then measured over time by a lithium-sensitive electrode attached to a peripheral arterial catheter. Lithium dilution has been shown to be reliable compared with the pulmonary artery catheter[10,11] and to be precise.[12]

The arterial pressure waveform analysis with the LiDCOplus, which uses the PulseCO algorithm, is the same as for the LiDCOrapid device and is detailed later. Note that the use of lithium is not authorized in all countries.

Uncalibrated Devices

All these devices share the advantage of not requiring calibration by thermodilution. The technique they use for pressure waveform analysis differs slightly between devices.

FloTrac/Vigileo

With this system, stroke volume is estimated as:

$$SV = K \times \text{pulsatility}$$

where K is a constant that quantifies arterial resistance and compliance.

K is estimated from the morphometric data of the patient and is based on the method described by Langewouters and colleagues[13] and supported by a large database of pressure tracings recorded in hyperdynamic and vasoplegic patients.[14] The estimation is based on K and the arterial pulsatility. The device provides the starting value of K. Then, K is automatically adapted every 60 seconds by taking into account some geometric properties of the arterial pressure curve, such as skewness and kurtosis. Pulsatility is estimated from the standard deviations of pulse pressure.

In practice, the device consists of a standard arterial catheter and a standard arterial line that is connected to a disposable specific pressure transducer (FloTrac). The pressure transducer is connected to the Vigileo device, which performs analysis and displays cardiac output.

ProAQT/Pulsioflex

Like the FloTrac/Vigileo system, the more recent ProAQT/Pulsioflex does not need any external calibration of pressure waveform analysis. Nevertheless, the main distinction of this device is that the initial value of cardiac output from which the pulse contour analysis is started is not estimated by pulse contour analysis but by an innovative proprietary algorithm that performs an autocalibration. It uses the biometric values (age, height, and weight) as well as mean arterial pressure and heart rate. The cardiac output value is inferred from a statistical analysis of these data; this analysis is confidential and is not a Windkessel model. After the initial estimation of cardiac output, the ProAQT/Pulsioflex performs pulse contour analysis with a method similar to that of the PiCCO.

With the ProAQT/Pulsioflex, an automatic autocalibration of cardiac output can also be done at any time by just clicking a button. This autocalibration is supposed to reduce the drift that may have occurred since the previous estimation. In addition, it is also possible to manually enter a value for cardiac output measured by another technique (eg, echocardiography). The pulse contour analysis then starts from this external calibration value.

In practice, the device works with a standard arterial catheter and arterial line, which are connected to a specific disposable pressure transducer (ProAQT), which is connected to the monitor (Pulsioflex).

LiDCOrapid

This device is an evolution of the LiDCOplus that does not require any calibration. Pressure waveform analysis uses the same PulseCO algorithm as the LiDCOplus (described earlier). The PulseCO algorithm is based on the principles of conservation of mass and power and is not based on a Windkessel approach. Stroke volume is calculated from an analysis of the stroke volume–induced pulsatile change in the pressure waveform.

In addition, the arterial compliance is inferred from the age, height, and weight of the patient through established nomograms. The system does not need any calibration but, as with the ProAQT/Pulsioflex, it is possible to manually enter a value of cardiac output measured by an independent technique.

Pressure recording analytical method

The pressure recording analytical method (PRAM) is embedded in the MostCare device. With this method, the arterial pressure waveform analysis is based on the complex theory of perturbations. The estimation of cardiac output is grossly based on the area under the arterial pressure curve, on the analytical description of the arterial pressure waveform, and on the instantaneous acceleration of the arterial vessel cross-sectional area.

With this technique, the arterial impedance is only estimated by the characteristics of the arterial pressure curve, with no need for any calibration and independently from the morphometric data of the patient.[15]

RELIABILITY OF ARTERIAL PRESSURE WAVEFORM ANALYSIS DEVICES

The validation of devices providing a pressure-based estimation of cardiac output has been the purpose of several studies. It is difficult to summarize them, because they have provided heterogeneous results. Moreover, the technique used as the reference (eg, the pulmonary artery catheter) has its own limitations. An example of this is shown in **Fig. 2**, which is adapted from a study in which the pulmonary artery catheter showed bias and limits of agreement that were similar to those of some pulse waveform analysis devices (see **Fig. 2**).[16] Nevertheless, this article aims to clarify the validation of different devices.

Calibrated Devices

PiCCO

The validation of the pulse contour analysis of the PiCCO device has been performed by some clinical studies comparing it with the pulmonary artery catheter, which was used as a reference. Overall, these studies show that this reliability is acceptable.[3,9,17–23] Note that, as stated earlier, the closer the measurement from a previous calibration, the better the reliability.[9]

The validation of a device measuring cardiac output should be based not only on its accuracy, which is its ability to provide a value that is close to the true value, but also on its precision, which is the ability to provide values that are close to each other. In

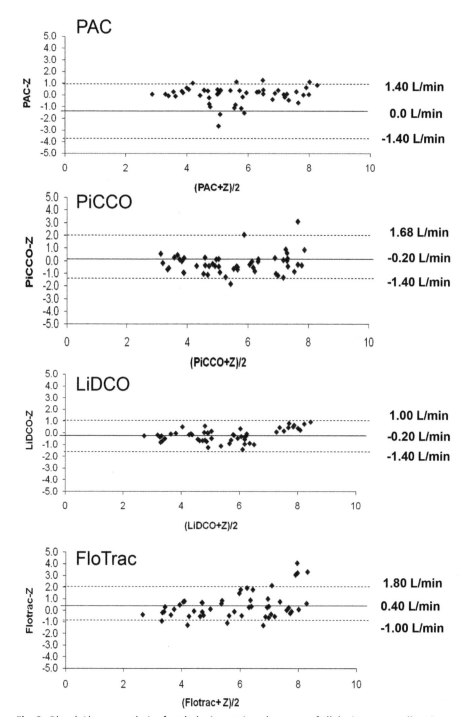

Fig. 2. Bland-Altman analysis of each device against the mean of all devices across all patients, wherein pulmonary arterial catheter (PAC), thermodilution cardiac output, and continuous cardiac output measured by the PAC are pooled to be 1 variable (Z-statistic). Solid line, mean difference (bias); dotted line, limits of agreement (bias ± 1.96 standard deviation). (*From* Hadian M, Kim HK, Severyn DA, et al. Cross-comparison of cardiac output trending accuracy of LiDCO, PiCCO, FloTrac and pulmonary artery catheters. Crit Care 2010;14:R212.)

this regard, the coefficient of variation of pulse contour analysis with the PiCCO is less than 2%,[9] which means that, if the patient's condition is stable, even small changes in cardiac output detected by pulse contour analysis should be considered as reliable.[24]

LiDCOplus

Reliability of the LiDCOplus device compared with thermodilution methods has been reported by concordant studies.[25–27] Because of its specific PulseCO algorithm, the estimation of cardiac output by the LiDCOplus is supposed to be less sensitive to changes in the morphology of the arterial curve than pulse contour analysis, especially in cases of vasopressor administration. The technique is also supposed to be less sensitive to arterial line damping than other pulse wave analysis techniques. Nevertheless, these potential advantages have not been shown until now.

Volumeview/EV1000

The reliability of pulse contour analysis measured by the more recent VolumeView/EV1000 has so far been shown by only 1 study,[28] which also reported a good tracking ability compared with transpulmonary thermodilution.

Overall, it is reasonable to consider that the calibrated pulse contour analysis systems are reliable to estimate cardiac output. This reliability is mostly related to the possibility to regularly reset the estimation with transpulmonary dilution, a technique that itself provides a reliable measurement of cardiac output. These calibrated devices have the disadvantage of requiring injections of cold boluses or lithium. With the PiCCO and VolumeView/EV1000 devices, such injections require a large-diameter arterial catheter, so these techniques cannot be described as minimally invasive.

Uncalibrated Devices

FloTrac/Vigileo

Results concerning the reliability of the uncalibrated devices are not as concordant as for the calibrated devices. The FloTrac/Vigileo, as the precursor of such devices, was the most studied. Although some studies reported good reliability,[14,29–34] some others found opposite results.[35–47]

One possible explanation for this discrepancy may concern the setting in which the studies were conducted. Overall, most of the studies showing good reliability of the FloTrac/Vigileo were conducted in perioperative settings,[29–31,33] even though poor results were also obtained in such patients.[48] The poorest results were obtained in critically ill patients[40,41,43,47] or patients undergoing liver surgery[36–39,44–46] (ie, in patients with large changes in vasomotor tone). The reliability of the FloTrac/Vigileo seems to decrease if the vasomotor tone changes to a large extent.[35,38,41–43] Note that the reliability of a cardiac output monitoring device depends not only on its ability to provide a reliable absolute value of cardiac output but also on its ability to track changes in cardiac output.

For instance, Monnet and colleagues[43] found that the reliability of the last version of the FloTrac/Vigileo was much poorer in tracking the changes in cardiac output when they were induced by changing the dose of norepinephrine than by administering a volume expansion. It was similarly reported that the reliability of the FloTrac/Vigileo was poor during liver transplant surgery and that the poorest results were obtained when the systemic vascular resistance changed to a large extent.[38] In some patients before surgical intervention, the FloTrac/Vigileo provided a good estimation of cardiac output compared with esophageal Doppler when preload was increased, whereas it was poor when the arterial tone was modified by ephedrine or phenylephrine.[42] The trending ability of the third version of the FloTrac/Vigileo during phenylephrine administration similarly was the lowest when the systemic vascular resistance was the highest.[49] Overall, the failure of uncalibrated pulse contour analysis may be related mainly to its inability to take into account changes in vascular tone.

All situations in which the arterial pressure waveform is abnormally modified are also at risk for unreliability of uncalibrated pulse contour analysis. This unreliability can arise in cases of dampening of the arterial pressure curve, which justifies careful checking of the arterial line when such devices are used. This unreliability can be related to air bubbles, blood clots in the arterial catheter, or kinking of the arterial catheter line.

Aortic valvular regurgitation[35] and stenosis[50] are other conditions in which pulse contour analysis by the FloTrac/Vigileo has been shown to have poor reliability, even though it could still reliably track the changes in cardiac output.[50] Such uncalibrated devices produced conflicting results with intra-aortic balloon pumps, some with acceptable[51] and others with unacceptable biases and limits of agreement.[35]

The reliability of the uncalibrated devices may also depend on the arterial site to which they are connected. Nevertheless, some results showed no[41,52] or minimal[53] differences between cardiac output values obtained from the femoral and the radial sites.

LiDCOrapid

The LiDCOrapid device has had less evaluation. In patients undergoing cardiac surgery, the estimation of cardiac output by pulse power analysis was influenced by the mean arterial pressure, yielding an unacceptable bias.[54] A high percentage error was also recently reported for this device compared with esophageal Doppler monitoring, associated with a bad trending ability.[55]

ProAQT/Pulsioflex

The recent ProAQT/Pulsioflex device still requires validation studies. In particular, these studies should investigate whether the autocalibration allowed by the ProAQT/Pulsioflex improves the measurement of cardiac output.

Pressure recording analytical method

The PRAM algorithm of the MostCare device has been investigated by only a few studies. In patients after cardiac surgery and with an intra-aortic balloon pump, this uncalibrated estimation of cardiac output was acceptable.[15] In septic patients receiving norepinephrine, and compared with the pulmonary artery catheter, the PRAM system showed an acceptable percentage of error.[56] This finding was also shown in cardiac surgical patients; even in those with an intra-aortic balloon pump[51,57,58] (ie, patients in whom pulse waveform analysis is usually considered inoperative). In contrast with these positive results, another study from a different group found a profound lack of agreement between PRAM and the pulmonary artery catheter, without any obvious explanation for this discrepancy.[59]

THE ADVANTAGE OF A REAL-TIME MONITORING OF CARDIAC OUTPUT WITH ARTERIAL PRESSURE WAVEFORM ANALYSIS

The most important advantage of the arterial pressure waveform contour analysis technique is that it provides a real-time measurement of cardiac output because it is based on a measurement of stroke volume from beat to beat. This real-time measurement is useful in 2 ways.

Stroke Volume Variation

All the arterial pressure waveform analysis devices measure the percentage of variation of stroke volume over time. This variation within the respiratory cycle is associated with preload reserve, based on the same principle as pulse pressure variation.[60] Even though stroke volume and pulse pressure variations are not exactly the same,[61,62] stroke volume variation has regularly been shown to predict fluid responsiveness as reliably as pulse pressure variation.[63–80]

Note that stroke volume variation has the same limitations as pulse pressure variation.[81] It cannot be used to predict fluid responsiveness in cases of spontaneous breathing activity, cardiac arrhythmias, low tidal volume and low lung compliance,[82] and open chest conditions.

Short-term Changes in Cardiac Output

Arterial pressure waveform analysis is particularly suitable for assessing changes in cardiac output occurring on a very short time scale. Note that this is not the case for the semicontinuous thermodilution by the pulmonary artery catheter, which reflects only the changes in cardiac output that occurred during the last few minutes.

For instance, arterial pressure waveform analysis is particularly suitable for assessing the effects of the passive leg raising test[24,63,64,82–84] or of the end-expiratory occlusion test,[24,82,85] which exert their hemodynamic effects on periods of time that are too short to use a dilution method.

CONTEXT OF USE OF ARTERIAL PRESSURE WAVEFORM ANALYSIS DEVICES
Uncalibrated Devices

The typical indication for the uncalibrated pulse contour analysis devices is the monitoring of surgical interventions in high-risk surgical patients. First, as detailed earlier, it is in this context that the reliability of cardiac output measurement by such devices has been found to be the best. The low invasiveness of the uncalibrated devices is particularly appropriate for these patients with a low risk of complications during surgery.

The poor results obtained during liver surgery[36–39,44–46] suggest that the uncalibrated devices should not be used during this type of surgery, which is associated with large changes in vascular tone. Also, during cardiac surgery, hemodynamic evaluation by uncalibrated pulse contour analysis devices is likely to be too limited. In addition, the measurement of cardiac output, along with stroke volume variation, fits the requirement of hemodynamic monitoring during surgery, which is to alert the anesthesiologist of a hemodynamic impairment.[86]

In surgery for high-risk patients, hemodynamic monitoring by uncalibrated devices attached to a therapeutic protocol has been found to decrease the risk of complications, either with the PiCCO[87] or the Vigileo.[88,89] This finding reinforces the message that a preemptive hemodynamic intervention improves the postoperative outcome of such patients.[90]

Calibrated Devices

These devices are likely more indicated in critically ill patients. In these patients, who often receive vasopressors and in whom the vasomotor tone is unstable, external calibration reduces the errors in cardiac output measurement by pulse contour analysis related to changes in vasomotor tone. The invasiveness of such devices is more acceptable in critically ill patients than in surgical patients because of the greater severity of their illnesses, even though the rate complications related to the calibrated pulse contour analysis devices is low.[8] In addition, in this context the intensivist may be interested in the other hemodynamic variables that pulmonary thermodilution provides besides pulse contour analysis.[91]

PULSE CONTOUR ANALYSIS FROM A NONINVASIVE ARTERIAL PRESSURE CURVE

The Nexfin device (Edwards Lifesciences, Irvine, CA) provides a noninvasive estimation of the arterial pressure curve and uses it to compute cardiac output.

Tracing of the Noninvasive Arterial Curve

The Nexfin device allows a continuous estimation of the arterial pressure curve through the volume-clamp method.[92] For this purpose, the device includes an inflatable cuff that is wrapped around a finger. It also includes a photoplethysmographic device that measures the diameter of the finger arteries. At each systole, the photoplethysmographic device senses the increase of the finger arteries' diameters. A fast servo-controlled system immediately inflates the cuff in order to keep the arteries' diameters constant. Therefore, cuff pressure reflects the arterial pressure. Its continuous measurement allows estimation of the arterial pressure curve.

This measurement of arterial pressure by Nexfin has been largely validated for measuring arterial pressure.[93–100]

Estimation of Cardiac Output

To estimate cardiac output, the device uses a pulse contour waveform analysis. With this device, aortic impedance is determined from a 3-element Windkessel model that incorporates the influence of nonlinear effects of arterial pressure and of the patient's age, height, weight, and gender on aortic mechanical properties.[101] The Nexfin method was developed on a database including invasive and noninvasive arterial pressures together with thermodilution cardiac output values.

The reliability of this estimation of cardiac output has provided discrepant results, with both positive[94,102–108] and negative studies.[100,109,110]

The most plausible hypothesis explaining this discrepancy is the difference in the population of interest. The studies that showed a better reliability of the Nexfin were conducted in the operating theater,[102,103] in patients having cardiac surgery after discontinuation of mechanical ventilation and inotropes,[94] in patients undergoing resynchronization therapy,[105] in an echocardiography laboratory,[104] or in healthy subjects.[107] By contrast, the studies reporting unreliability of the technique[100,109] included critically ill patients, most with septic shock. In such patients, poor finger perfusion likely impedes the correct assessment of the finger pressure curve by the volume-clamp method, which includes an analysis of the finger photoplethysmographic signal. This limitation suggests that such a device is more suitable for the operating theater than for intensive care units.

SUMMARY

The number of less invasive devices monitoring cardiac output using a pressure-based estimation of cardiac output has increased during recent years. The low invasiveness of such systems, which is a particular advantage in operating theaters, seems to be counterbalanced by a reliability that is lower than for more invasive devices. This lower reliability applies particularly in comparisons of calibrated and uncalibrated pulse contour analyzing devices. Technological improvement in these recently developed devices may reduce this limitation of less invasive devices.

REFERENCES

1. Richard C, Monnet X, Teboul JL. Pulmonary artery catheter monitoring in 2011. Curr Opin Crit Care 2011;17:296–302.

2. Wesseling KH, Jansen JR, Settels JJ, et al. Computation of aortic flow from pressure in humans using a nonlinear, three-element model. J Appl Physiol (1985) 1993;74:2566–73.

3. Goedje O, Hoeke K, Lichtwarck-Aschoff M, et al. Continuous cardiac output by femoral arterial thermodilution calibrated pulse contour analysis: comparison with pulmonary arterial thermodilution. Crit Care Med 1999;27: 2407–12.

4. Reuter DA, Huang C, Edrich T, et al. Cardiac output monitoring using indicator-dilution techniques: basics, limits, and perspectives. Anesth Analg 2010;110: 799–811.

5. Monnet X, Persichini R, Ktari M, et al. Precision of the transpulmonary thermodilution measurements. Crit Care 2011;15:R204.

6. Monnet X, Teboul JL. Clinical utility of extravascular lung water measurements. In: Vincent JL, editor. Yearbook of intensive care and emergency medicine. Berlin; Heidelberg (Germany); New York: Springer-Verlag; 2009. p. 433–42.

7. Jabot J, Monnet X, Lamia B, et al. Cardiac function index provided by transpulmonary thermodilution behaves as an indicator of left ventricular systolic function. Crit Care Med 2009;37:2913–8.

8. Belda FJ, Aguilar G, Teboul JL, et al. Complications related to less-invasive haemodynamic monitoring. Br J Anaesth 2011;106:482–6.

9. Hamzaoui O, Monnet X, Richard C, et al. Effects of changes in vascular tone on the agreement between pulse contour and transpulmonary thermodilution cardiac output measurements within an up to 6-hour calibration-free period. Crit Care Med 2008;36:434–40.

10. Linton R, Band D, O'Brien T, et al. Lithium dilution cardiac output measurement: a comparison with thermodilution. Crit Care Med 1997;25:1796–800.

11. Kurita T, Morita K, Kato S, et al. Comparison of the accuracy of the lithium dilution technique with the thermodilution technique for measurement of cardiac output. Br J Anaesth 1997;79:770–5.

12. Cecconi M, Dawson D, Grounds RM, et al. Lithium dilution cardiac output measurement in the critically ill patient: determination of precision of the technique. Intensive Care Med 2009;35:498–504.

13. Langewouters GJ, Wesseling KH, Goedhard WJ. The static elastic properties of 45 human thoracic and 20 abdominal aortas in vitro and the parameters of a new model. J Biomech 1984;17:425–35.

14. De Backer D, Marx G, Tan A, et al. Arterial pressure-based cardiac output monitoring: a multicenter validation of the third-generation software in septic patients. Intensive Care Med 2011;37:233–40.

15. Romano SM, Pistolesi M. Assessment of cardiac output from systemic arterial pressure in humans. Crit Care Med 2002;30:1834–41.

16. Hadian M, Kim HK, Severyn DA, et al. Cross-comparison of cardiac output trending accuracy of LiDCO, PiCCO, FloTrac and pulmonary artery catheters. Crit Care 2010;14:R212.

17. Bein B, Worthmann F, Tonner PH, et al. Comparison of esophageal Doppler, pulse contour analysis, and real-time pulmonary artery thermodilution for the continuous measurement of cardiac output. J Cardiothorac Vasc Anesth 2004; 18:185–9.

18. Buhre W, Weyland A, Kazmaier S, et al. Comparison of cardiac output assessed by pulse-contour analysis and thermodilution in patients undergoing minimally invasive direct coronary artery bypass grafting. J Cardiothorac Vasc Anesth 1999;13:437–40.

19. Felbinger TW, Reuter DA, Eltzschig HK, et al. Cardiac index measurements during rapid preload changes: a comparison of pulmonary artery thermodilution with arterial pulse contour analysis. J Clin Anesth 2005;17:241–8.

20. Felbinger TW, Reuter DA, Eltzschig HK, et al. Comparison of pulmonary arterial thermodilution and arterial pulse contour analysis: evaluation of a new algorithm. J Clin Anesth 2002;14:296–301.

21. Godje O, Hoke K, Goetz AE, et al. Reliability of a new algorithm for continuous cardiac output determination by pulse-contour analysis during hemodynamic instability. Crit Care Med 2002;30:52–8.

22. Rodig G, Prasser C, Keyl C, et al. Continuous cardiac output measurement: pulse contour analysis vs thermodilution technique in cardiac surgical patients. Br J Anaesth 1999;82:525–30.

23. Zollner C, Haller M, Weis M, et al. Beat-to-beat measurement of cardiac output by intravascular pulse contour analysis: a prospective criterion standard study in patients after cardiac surgery. J Cardiothorac Vasc Anesth 2000;14:125–9.

24. Monnet X, Osman D, Ridel C, et al. Predicting volume responsiveness by using the end-expiratory occlusion in mechanically ventilated intensive care unit patients. Crit Care Med 2009;37:951–6.

25. Costa MG, Della Rocca G, Chiarandini P, et al. Continuous and intermittent cardiac output measurement in hyperdynamic conditions: pulmonary artery catheter vs. lithium dilution technique. Intensive Care Med 2008;34:257–63.

26. Missant C, Rex S, Wouters PF. Accuracy of cardiac output measurements with pulse contour analysis (PulseCO) and Doppler echocardiography during off-pump coronary artery bypass grafting. Eur J Anaesthesiol 2008;25:243–8.

27. Pittman J, Bar-Yosef S, SumPing J, et al. Continuous cardiac output monitoring with pulse contour analysis: a comparison with lithium indicator dilution cardiac output measurement. Crit Care Med 2005;33:2015–21.

28. Bendjelid K, Marx G, Kiefer N, et al. Performance of a new pulse contour method for continuous cardiac output monitoring: validation in critically ill patients. Br J Anaesth 2013;111:573–9.

29. Button D, Weibel L, Reuthebuch O, et al. Clinical evaluation of the FloTrac/Vigileo system and two established continuous cardiac output monitoring devices in patients undergoing cardiac surgery. Br J Anaesth 2007;99:329–36.

30. Cannesson M, Attof Y, Rosamel P, et al. Comparison of FloTrac cardiac output monitoring system in patients undergoing coronary artery bypass grafting with pulmonary artery cardiac output measurements. Eur J Anaesthesiol 2007;24:832–9.

31. de Waal EE, Kalkman CJ, Rex S, et al. Validation of a new arterial pulse contour-based cardiac output device. Crit Care Med 2007;35:1904–9.

32. Mayer J, Boldt J, Schollhorn T, et al. Semi-invasive monitoring of cardiac output by a new device using arterial pressure waveform analysis: a comparison with intermittent pulmonary artery thermodilution in patients undergoing cardiac surgery. Br J Anaesth 2007;98:176–82.

33. Senn A, Button D, Zollinger A, et al. Assessment of cardiac output changes using a modified FloTrac/Vigileo algorithm in cardiac surgery patients. Crit Care 2009;13:R32.

34. McLean AS, Huang SJ, Kot M, et al. Comparison of cardiac output measurements in critically ill patients: FloTrac/Vigileo vs transthoracic Doppler echocardiography. Anaesth Intensive Care 2011;39:590–8.

35. Lorsomradee S, Cromheecke S, De Hert SG. Uncalibrated arterial pulse contour analysis versus continuous thermodilution technique: effects of alterations in arterial waveform. J Cardiothorac Vasc Anesth 2007;21:636–43.

36. Biancofiore G, Critchley LA, Lee A, et al. Evaluation of an uncalibrated arterial pulse contour cardiac output monitoring system in cirrhotic patients undergoing liver surgery. Br J Anaesth 2009;102:47–54.

37. Della Rocca G, Costa MG, Chiarandini P, et al. Arterial pulse cardiac output agreement with thermodilution in patients in hyperdynamic conditions. J Cardiothorac Vasc Anesth 2008;22:681–7.

38. Biais M, Nouette-Gaulain K, Cottenceau V, et al. Cardiac output measurement in patients undergoing liver transplantation: pulmonary artery catheter versus uncalibrated arterial pressure waveform analysis. Anesth Analg 2008;106:1480–6.

39. Krejci V, Vannucci A, Abbas A, et al. Comparison of calibrated and uncalibrated arterial pressure-based cardiac output monitors during orthotopic liver transplantation. Liver Transpl 2010;16:773–82.

40. Junttila EK, Koskenkari JK, Ohtonen PP, et al. Uncalibrated arterial pressure waveform analysis for cardiac output monitoring is biased by low peripheral resistance in patients with intracranial haemorrhage. Br J Anaesth 2011;107: 581–6.

41. Monnet X, Anguel N, Naudin B, et al. Arterial pressure-based cardiac output in septic patients: different accuracy of pulse contour and uncalibrated pressure waveform devices. Crit Care 2010;14:R109.

42. Meng L, Phuong Tran N, Alexander BS, et al. The impact of phenylephrine, ephedrine, and increased preload on third-generation Vigileo-FloTrac and esophageal Doppler cardiac output measurements. Anesth Analg 2011;113: 751–7.

43. Monnet X, Anguel N, Jozwiak M, et al. Third-generation FloTrac/Vigileo does not reliably track the changes in cardiac output induced by norepinephrine in critically ill patients. Br J Anaesth 2012;108:615–22.

44. Biancofiore G, Critchley LA, Lee A, et al. Evaluation of a new software version of the FloTrac/Vigileo (version 3.02) and a comparison with previous data in cirrhotic patients undergoing liver transplant surgery. Anesth Analg 2011;113: 515–22.

45. Su BC, Tsai YF, Chen CY, et al. Cardiac output derived from arterial pressure waveform analysis in patients undergoing liver transplantation: validity of a third-generation device. Transplant Proc 2012;44:424–8.

46. Tsai YF, Su BC, Lin CC, et al. Cardiac output derived from arterial pressure waveform analysis: validation of the third-generation software in patients undergoing orthotopic liver transplantation. Transplant Proc 2012;44:433–7.

47. Metzelder S, Coburn M, Fries M, et al. Performance of cardiac output measurement derived from arterial pressure waveform analysis in patients requiring high-dose vasopressor therapy. Br J Anaesth 2011;106:776–84.

48. Desebbe O, Henaine R, Keller G, et al. Ability of the third-generation FloTrac/Vigileo software to track changes in cardiac output in cardiac surgery patients: a polar plot approach. J Cardiothorac Vasc Anesth 2013;27:1122–7.

49. Suehiro K, Tanaka K, Funao T, et al. Systemic vascular resistance has an impact on the reliability of the Vigileo-FloTrac system in measuring cardiac output and tracking cardiac output changes. Br J Anaesth 2013;111:170–7.

50. Petzoldt M, Riedel C, Braeunig J, et al. Stroke volume determination using transcardiopulmonary thermodilution and arterial pulse contour analysis in severe aortic valve disease. Intensive Care Med 2013;39:601–11.

51. Scolletta S, Franchi F, Taccone FS, et al. An uncalibrated pulse contour method to measure cardiac output during aortic counterpulsation. Anesth Analg 2011; 113:1389–95.
52. Vasdev S, Chauhan S, Choudhury M, et al. Arterial pressure waveform derived cardiac output FloTrac/Vigileo system (third generation software): comparison of two monitoring sites with the thermodilution cardiac output. J Clin Monit Comput 2012;26:115–20.
53. Schramm S, Albrecht E, Frascarolo P, et al. Validity of an arterial pressure waveform analysis device: does the puncture site play a role in the agreement with intermittent pulmonary artery catheter thermodilution measurements? J Cardiothorac Vasc Anesth 2010;24:250–6.
54. Broch O, Renner J, Hocker J, et al. Uncalibrated pulse power analysis fails to reliably measure cardiac output in patients undergoing coronary artery bypass surgery. Crit Care 2011;15:R76.
55. Nordstrom J, Hallsjo-Sander C, Shore R, et al. Stroke volume optimization in elective bowel surgery: a comparison between pulse power wave analysis (LiDCOrapid) and oesophageal Doppler (CardioQ). Br J Anaesth 2013;110:374–80.
56. Franchi F, Silvestri R, Cubattoli L, et al. Comparison between an uncalibrated pulse contour method and thermodilution technique for cardiac output estimation in septic patients. Br J Anaesth 2011;107:202–8.
57. Zangrillo A, Maj G, Monaco F, et al. Cardiac index validation using the pressure recording analytic method in unstable patients. J Cardiothorac Vasc Anesth 2010;24:265–9.
58. Barile L, Landoni G, Pieri M, et al. Cardiac index assessment by the pressure recording analytic method in critically ill unstable patients after cardiac surgery. J Cardiothorac Vasc Anesth 2013;27:1108–13.
59. Paarmann H, Groesdonk HV, Sedemund-Adib B, et al. Lack of agreement between pulmonary arterial thermodilution cardiac output and the pressure recording analytical method in postoperative cardiac surgery patients. Br J Anaesth 2011;106:475–81.
60. Monnet X, Teboul JL. Assessment of volume responsiveness during mechanical ventilation: recent advances. Crit Care 2013;17:217.
61. de Wilde RB, Geerts BF, van den Berg PC, et al. A comparison of stroke volume variation measured by the LiDCOplus and FloTrac-Vigileo system. Anaesthesia 2009;64:1004–9.
62. Pinsky MR. Functional hemodynamic monitoring. Intensive Care Med 2002;28: 386–8.
63. Monnet X, Dres M, Ferre A, et al. Prediction of fluid responsiveness by a continuous non-invasive assessment of arterial pressure in critically ill patients: comparison with four other dynamic indices. Br J Anaesth 2012;109:330–8.
64. Monnet X, Guerin L, Jozwiak M, et al. Pleth variability index is a weak predictor of fluid responsiveness in patients receiving norepinephrine. Br J Anaesth 2013; 110:207–13.
65. Rex S, Schalte G, Schroth S, et al. Limitations of arterial pulse pressure variation and left ventricular stroke volume variation in estimating cardiac pre-load during open heart surgery. Acta Anaesthesiol Scand 2007;51:1258–67.
66. Marx G, Cope T, McCrossan L, et al. Assessing fluid responsiveness by stroke volume variation in mechanically ventilated patients with severe sepsis. Eur J Anaesthesiol 2004;21:132–8.
67. Vos JJ, Kalmar AF, Struys MM, et al. Comparison of arterial pressure and plethysmographic waveform-based dynamic preload variables in assessing

fluid responsiveness and dynamic arterial tone in patients undergoing major hepatic resection. Br J Anaesth 2013;110:940–6.

68. Trepte CJ, Eichhorn V, Haas SA, et al. Comparison of an automated respiratory systolic variation test with dynamic preload indicators to predict fluid responsiveness after major surgery. Br J Anaesth 2013;111:736–42.

69. Biais M, Nouette-Gaulain K, Cottenceau V, et al. Uncalibrated pulse contour-derived stroke volume variation predicts fluid responsiveness in mechanically ventilated patients undergoing liver transplantation. Br J Anaesth 2008;101:761–8.

70. Berkenstadt H, Margalit N, Hadani M, et al. Stroke volume variation as a predictor of fluid responsiveness in patients undergoing brain surgery. Anesth Analg 2001;92:984–9.

71. Yang SY, Shim JK, Song Y, et al. Validation of pulse pressure variation and corrected flow time as predictors of fluid responsiveness in patients in the prone position. Br J Anaesth 2013;110:713–20.

72. Hofer CK, Senn A, Weibel L, et al. Assessment of stroke volume variation for prediction of fluid responsiveness using the modified FloTrac and PiCCOplus system. Crit Care 2008;12:R82.

73. Reuter DA, Kirchner A, Felbinger TW, et al. Usefulness of left ventricular stroke volume variation to assess fluid responsiveness in patients with reduced cardiac function. Crit Care Med 2003;31:1399–404.

74. Derichard A, Robin E, Tavernier B, et al. Automated pulse pressure and stroke volume variations from radial artery: evaluation during major abdominal surgery. Br J Anaesth 2009;103:678–84.

75. Hofer CK, Muller SM, Furrer L, et al. Stroke volume and pulse pressure variation for prediction of fluid responsiveness in patients undergoing off-pump coronary artery bypass grafting. Chest 2005;128:848–54.

76. Cannesson M, Musard H, Desebbe O, et al. The ability of stroke volume variations obtained with Vigileo/FloTrac system to monitor fluid responsiveness in mechanically ventilated patients. Anesth Analg 2009;108:513–7.

77. Wiesenack C, Fiegl C, Keyser A, et al. Assessment of fluid responsiveness in mechanically ventilated cardiac surgical patients. Eur J Anaesthesiol 2005;22:658–65.

78. Reuter DA, Felbinger TW, Schmidt C, et al. Stroke volume variations for assessment of cardiac responsiveness to volume loading in mechanically ventilated patients after cardiac surgery. Intensive Care Med 2002;28:392–8.

79. Biais M, Bernard O, Ha JC, et al. Abilities of pulse pressure variations and stroke volume variations to predict fluid responsiveness in prone position during scoliosis surgery. Br J Anaesth 2010;104:407–13.

80. Preisman S, Kogan S, Berkenstadt H, et al. Predicting fluid responsiveness in patients undergoing cardiac surgery: functional haemodynamic parameters including the respiratory systolic variation test and static preload indicators. Br J Anaesth 2005;95:746–55.

81. Marik PE, Monnet X, Teboul JL. Hemodynamic parameters to guide fluid therapy. Ann Intensive Care 2011;1:1.

82. Monnet X, Bleibtreu A, Ferré A, et al. Passive leg raising and end-expiratory occlusion tests perform better than pulse pressure variation in patients with low respiratory system compliance. Crit Care Med 2012;40:152–7.

83. Monnet X, Bataille A, Magalhaes E, et al. End-tidal carbon dioxide is better than arterial pressure for predicting volume responsiveness by the passive leg raising test. Intensive Care Med 2013;39:93–100.

84. Monnet X, Jabot J, Maizel J, et al. Norepinephrine increases cardiac preload and reduces preload dependency assessed by passive leg raising in septic shock patients. Crit Care Med 2011;39:689–94.
85. Silva S, Jozwiak M, Teboul JL, et al. End-expiratory occlusion test predicts preload responsiveness independently of positive end-expiratory pressure during acute respiratory distress syndrome. Crit Care Med 2013;41:1692–701.
86. Vincent JL, Rhodes A, Perel A, et al. Clinical review: update on hemodynamic monitoring - a consensus of 16. Crit Care 2011;15:229.
87. Salzwedel C, Puig J, Carstens A, et al. Perioperative goal-directed hemodynamic therapy based on radial arterial pulse pressure variation and continuous cardiac index trending reduces postoperative complications after major abdominal surgery: a multi-center, prospective, randomized study. Crit Care 2013;17:R191.
88. Benes J, Chytra I, Altmann P, et al. Intraoperative fluid optimization using stroke volume variation in high risk surgical patients: results of prospective randomized study. Crit Care 2010;14:R118.
89. Cecconi M, Fasano N, Langiano N, et al. Goal-directed haemodynamic therapy during elective total hip arthroplasty under regional anaesthesia. Crit Care 2011; 15:R132.
90. Hamilton MA, Cecconi M, Rhodes A. A systematic review and meta-analysis on the use of preemptive hemodynamic intervention to improve postoperative outcomes in moderate and high-risk surgical patients. Anesth Analg 2011;112: 1392–402.
91. Sakka SG, Reuter DA, Perel A. The transpulmonary thermodilution technique. J Clin Monit Comput 2012;26:347–53.
92. Penaz J. Photoelectric measurement of blood pressure, volume and flow in the finger. Digest of the 10th International Conference on Medical and Biological Engineering. Dresden, 1973.
93. Hofhuizen CM, Lemson J, Hemelaar AE, et al. Continuous non-invasive finger arterial pressure monitoring reflects intra-arterial pressure changes in children undergoing cardiac surgery. Br J Anaesth 2010;105:493–500.
94. Bogert LW, Wesseling KH, Schraa O, et al. Pulse contour cardiac output derived from non-invasive arterial pressure in cardiovascular disease. Anaesthesia 2010;65:1119–25.
95. Broch O, Bein B, Gruenewald M, et al. Accuracy of the pleth variability index to predict fluid responsiveness depends on the perfusion index. Acta Anaesthesiol Scand 2011;55:686–93.
96. Eeftinck Schattenkerk DW, van Lieshout JJ, van den Meiracker AH, et al. Nexfin noninvasive continuous blood pressure validated against Riva-Rocci/Korotkoff. Am J Hypertens 2009;22:378–83.
97. Martina JR, Westerhof BE, van Goudoever J, et al. Noninvasive continuous arterial blood pressure monitoring with Nexfin. Anesthesiology 2012;116(5): 1092–103.
98. Nowak RM, Sen A, Garcia AJ, et al. Noninvasive continuous or intermittent blood pressure and heart rate patient monitoring in the ED. Am J Emerg Med 2011;29: 782–9.
99. Maggi R, Viscardi V, Furukawa T, et al. Non-invasive continuous blood pressure monitoring of tachycardic episodes during interventional electrophysiology. Europace 2010;12:1616–22.
100. Monnet X, Picard F, Lidzborski E, et al. The estimation of cardiac output by the Nexfin device is of poor reliability for tracking the effects of a fluid challenge. Crit Care 2012;16:R212.

101. Westerhof N, Elzinga G, Sipkema P. An artificial arterial system for pumping hearts. J Appl Physiol 1971;31:776–81.
102. Broch O, Renner J, Gruenewald M, et al. A comparison of the Nexfin® and transcardiopulmonary thermodilution to estimate cardiac output during coronary artery surgery. Anaesthesia 2012;67:377–83.
103. Chen G, Meng L, Alexander B, et al. Comparison of noninvasive cardiac output measurements using the Nexfin monitoring device and the esophageal Doppler. J Clin Anesth 2012;24:275–83.
104. van der Spoel AG, Voogel AJ, Folkers A, et al. Comparison of noninvasive continuous arterial waveform analysis (Nexfin) with transthoracic Doppler echocardiography for monitoring of cardiac output. J Clin Anesth 2012;24:304–9.
105. van Geldorp IE, Delhaas T, Hermans B, et al. Comparison of a non-invasive arterial pulse contour technique and echo Doppler aorta velocity-time integral on stroke volume changes in optimization of cardiac resynchronization therapy. Europace 2011;13:87–95.
106. Stover JF, Stocker R, Lenherr R, et al. Noninvasive cardiac output and blood pressure monitoring cannot replace an invasive monitoring system in critically ill patients. BMC Anesthesiol 2009;9:6.
107. Bartels SA, Stok WJ, Bezemer R, et al. Noninvasive cardiac output monitoring during exercise testing: Nexfin pulse contour analysis compared to an inert gas rebreathing method and respired gas analysis. J Clin Monit Comput 2011;25:315–21.
108. Bubenek-Turconi SI, Craciun M, Miclea I, et al. Noninvasive continuous cardiac output by the Nexfin before and after preload-modifying maneuvers: a comparison with intermittent thermodilution cardiac output. Anesth Analg 2013;117: 366–72.
109. Fischer MO, Avram R, Carjaliu I, et al. Non-invasive continuous arterial pressure and cardiac index monitoring with Nexfin after cardiac surgery. Br J Anaesth 2012;109(4):514–21.
110. Taton O, Fagnoul D, De Backer D, et al. Evaluation of cardiac output in intensive care using a non-invasive arterial pulse contour technique (Nexfin(®)) compared with echocardiography. Anaesthesia 2013;68:917–23.

Bedside Ultrasonography for the Intensivist

Jose Cardenas-Garcia, MD*, Paul H. Mayo, MD

KEYWORDS

- Critical care ultrasonography • Critical care echocardiography
- Thoracic ultrasonography • Vascular ultrasonography • Abdominal ultrasonography

KEY POINTS

- Point-of-care ultrasonography is conceptually related to physical examination.
- The intensivist uses visual assessment, auscultation, and palpation on an ongoing basis to monitor their patient.
- Ultrasonography adds to traditional physical examination by allowing the intensivist to visualize the anatomy and function of the body in real time.

Videos of a normal parasternal long-axis view, a normal parasternal short-axis view, a normal apical 4-chamber view, a normal subcostal long-axis view, an inferior vena cava long longitudinal axis view, a severely reduced left ventricular systolic function, a moderately reduced left ventricular systolic function, a hyperdynamic left ventricular systolic function, a right ventricular pressure overload, acute cor pulmonale, a pericardial and pleural effusion, a pericardial tamponade, aortic stenosis, valvular vegetation, papillary muscle rupture, pleural effusion, lung sliding and A lines, lung pulse, lung point, B lines, a consolidation pattern, a noncompressible common femoral vein diagnostic of thrombus, a compressible common femoral vein and artery, a compressible common femoral vein at the level of the saphenous vein intake, a femoral vein at common femoral artery bifurcation, a fully compressible common femoral vein, a fully compressible superficial femoral vein, a fully compressible popliteal vein, FAST study of right side, FAST study of suprapubic area, FAST study of left side accompany this article at http:// www.criticalcare.theclinics.com/

Division of Pulmonary, Critical Care and Sleep Medicine, Hofstra North Shore LIJ School of Medicine, 410 Lakeville Road, Suite 107, New Hyde Park, NY 11042, USA
* Corresponding author. 410 Lakeville Road, Lake Success, NY 11042.
E-mail address: jdecardenasg@gmail.com

Crit Care Clin 31 (2015) 43–66
http://dx.doi.org/10.1016/j.ccc.2014.08.003   criticalcare.theclinics.com

INTRODUCTION

Critical care ultrasonography (CCUS) has utility for the diagnosis and management of critical illness. By definition, it is a bedside technique performed by the frontline clinician at point of care. Image acquisition, image interpretation, and application of the results to the clinical problem are the personal responsibility of the intensivist who is in charge of the case. This approach departs from the standard method of using ultrasonography in the intensive care unit (ICU), where radiology or cardiology service performs ultrasonography on a consultative basis.

Ultrasonography performed by the intensivist has advantages in comparison with the standard model.

- There is no delay in obtaining the study, thus avoiding the inevitable delay inherent in scheduling, performing, and interpreting the study when performed on a consultative basis.
- There is no disassociation between the individual who is interpreting the study and the clinical reality at the bedside. The intensivist performing the scan at the bedside can integrate knowledge of the history, physical, laboratory values, and other imaging results with the ultrasonography examination, whereas the off-line reader has a limited understanding of the case.
- The intensivist can repeat the examination as required to track the effects of therapy and the evolution of disease, and can perform limited or goal-directed examinations. The radiology and cardiology services have difficulty in performing repeated or limited studies.

Point-of-care ultrasonography is conceptually related to physical examination. The intensivist uses visual assessment, auscultation, and palpation on an ongoing basis to monitor the patient. Ultrasonography adds to traditional physical examination by allowing the intensivist to visualize the anatomy and function of the body in real time. Initial, repeated, and goal-directed ultrasonography is an extension of the physical examination that allows the intensivist to establish a diagnosis and monitor the condition of the patient on a regular basis.

THE COMPONENTS OF CRITICAL CARE ULTRASONOGRAPHY

The American College of Chest Physicians/La Société de Réanimation de Langue Française Statement on Competence in Critical Care Ultrasonography (ACCP/SRLF Statement) is a guide for the intensivist in setting goals of training.[1] The statement defines 5 modules of CCUS:

- Cardiac: basic and advanced levels
- Thoracic: lung and pleura
- Vascular access
- Vascular diagnostic: examination for deep venous thrombosis (DVT)
- Abdominal: screening examination

Another consensus statement that was sponsored by the major critical societies, The Expert Round Table on Ultrasound in ICU International Expert Statement on Training Standards for Critical Care Ultrasonography, offers guidance for the intensivist regarding the design of training.[2] The cognitive base of CCUS is available through review articles, textbooks, and original literature in the major journals. Training in image acquisition and interpretation is available in courses sponsored by the professional societies. Part of the training is performed at the bedside under the supervision of expert faculty, as scanning patients is not practical in standard course design. Competence in

CCUS also requires an autodidactic approach, particularly with reference to image acquisition. A major impetus to training will be the recent decision by the American Committee on Graduate Medical Education to require that knowledge of ultrasonography is a mandatory part of critical care fellowship training in the United States as from July 1, 2014.[3] This decision is in agreement with the Statement on Training Standards whereby the expert group established as an organizing principle that:

> Basic-level critical care echocardiography and general critical care ultrasound should be a required part of the training of every ICU physician.

Within a few years, all graduating fellows in the United States will be competent in CCUS; proficiency will become as standard as it is for airway management, bronchoscopy, or ventilator management.

EQUIPMENT REQUIREMENTS FOR CRITICAL CARE ULTRASONOGRAPHY

In general, modern portable ultrasonography machines have good image quality. The standard ICU machine is equipped with both a high-frequency (5.0–10 MHz) linear probe for vascular imaging and a low-frequency (1.0–5.0 MHz) phased-array probe for cardiac and thoracic imaging. Some machines are designed so that the cardiac probe can be configured for abdominal imaging so that it is a dual-purpose device, thus avoiding the need to purchase a third probe designed for abdominal scanning. In deciding on a machine for dedicated ICU use, the intensivist should consider the following questions:

- Durability: Is the machine drop and spill protected?
- Portability: Does the cart have a small profile; can the machine be removed from the cart and carried by hand?
- Ease of operation: Is the control surface simple and intuitive to operate?
- Transducer number: Is there a vascular and cardiac transducer; can the cardiac transducer be configured for use as an abdominal transducer (saving the cost of a third transducer)?
- Warranty cost: What is the cost of a full multiyear warranty; is it included in the machine acquisition cost, or is it an additional unanticipated cost?
- Reliability and service: What is the reliability of the device; does the company have an effective service network?
- Memory and archiving: Can the machine be interfaced with a wireless ICU-based image and report archiving system?

CARDIAC: BASIC AND ADVANCED LEVEL
Levels of Competence

The ACCP/SRLF Statement distinguishes between basic and advanced level critical care echocardiography (CCE).[1] Basic CCE uses a limited number of transthoracic echocardiography (TTE) views. Mastery of basic CCE is a key skill for all frontline critical care clinicians, and can be learned within a relatively short training period. Competence in advanced CCE requires a skill level comparable to a cardiology-trained echocardiographer in both TTE and transesophageal echocardiography (TEE), and entails a much longer duration of training in comparison with basic TTE.[4] This article focuses on basic CCE; other articles in this issue review some applications of advanced CCE.

Training in Basic Critical Care Echocardiography

Noncardiologists can achieve competence in basic CCE.[5] The requirements for training are not yet standardized; but the Statement on Training Standards recommends that training in basic CCE should include a minimum of 10 hours of course work (consisting of lectures, didactic cases, and image interpretation), and performance of at least 30 fully supervised TTE studies (including both image acquisition and interpretation).[2] These numbers offer guidance, but do not guarantee that the trainee is adequately trained. Competency-based testing following the completion of training offers assurance that the clinician has acquired the necessary skill. In addition to the ability to acquire and interpret the images, competence in basic CCE includes mastery of the cognitive elements of the field, including recognition of clinical syndromes with their associated basic CCE findings.

The Basic Critical Care Echocardiography Examination

The ACCP/SRLF Statement on Competence defines the basic CCE examination as including 5 standard views: the parasternal long-axis (PSL) view, the parasternal short-axis (PSS) view, the apical 4-chamber (AP4) view, the subcostal long-axis (SCL) view, and the inferior vena cava (IVC) longitudinal axis view. Several variations of the basic CCE examination have been proposed, with different acronyms; all have in common a limited number of views to rapidly assess cardiac anatomy and function in a goal-directed manner.

Owing to the nature of ICU patients, acquiring good-quality CCE views is often a challenge. The presence of equipment at the bedside, poor lighting conditions, electrodes, and monitor wires may make it difficult to achieve adequate probe position. The optimal position for the PSL, PSS, and AP4 views is with the patient in the left lateral decubitus position, which may be difficult to achieve in the critically ill patient. Image quality may be suboptimal in the edematous, obese, or muscular patient. Frequently some views may not be obtainable. For example, in the hyperinflated patient on ventilatory support, the SCL view may be the only one that yields a useful image. For this reason, it is important to attempt every view at every examination. This goal is best achieved by using a set scanning routine that is performed in the same sequence in every patient. It is common for the experienced examiner to use the following sequence: PSL, PSS, AP4, SCL, and IVC longitudinal.

With the current generation of portable ultrasonography machines, most medical ICU patients will yield adequate images using TTE. Image acquisition with TTE may not always be successful, because of body habitus or technical factors such as are present in the cardiothoracic surgical patient. In this situation, the use of TEE may be indicated.

The Five Standard Views of Basic Critical Care Echocardiography

Parasternal long-axis view

The transducer is placed in the left third to fifth intercostal space adjacent to the sternum with the orientation marker pointing toward the right shoulder of the patient (**Fig. 1**, Video 1). The tomographic plane is adjusted to line up the mitral valve (MV), aortic valve (AV), and the largest left ventricular (LV) area. Color Doppler may be used to examine for MV and AV regurgitation.

This view allows for assessment for pericardial effusion, LV/right ventricular (RV) size and function, left atrial (LA) size, septal kinetics, and valve anatomy. Pitfalls of this view include inaccurate assessment of LV size and function because of off-axis views (resulting in false end-systolic effacement), and underestimation or overestimation of regurgitant jets with color Doppler.

Parasternal short-axis midventricular level

From the PSL view, the transducer is rotated 90° clockwise without tilting or angling to obtain a cross-sectional view of the heart at the papillary muscle level with the orientation marker pointing toward the patient's left shoulder (**Fig. 2**, Video 2).

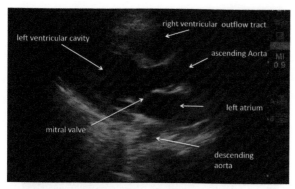

Fig. 1. Normal parasternal long-axis view.

This view allows for assessment for pericardial effusion, LV/RV size and function, and septal kinetics. Pitfalls of this view include inaccurate assessment of the LV geometry if an off-axis view is obtained, because overrotation of the transducer may result in false septal flattening.

Apical 4-chamber view
The probe is placed on the lower lateral chest with the orientation marker pointed toward the left shoulder of the patient (**Fig. 3**, Video 3). The tomographic plane is adjusted to bisect the anatomic apex of the left ventricle and the two atria.

This view is designed to assess the RV/LV ratio, LV/RV function, and for pericardial effusion. Pitfalls of this view include difficulty in obtaining an on-axis image, which can lead to inaccurate assessment of LV/RV function and RV/LV ratio.

Subcostal long-axis view
The probe is placed below the xiphoid process with the orientation marker pointing toward the 3 to 4 o'clock position, and the tomographic plane adjusted to bisect the left ventricle and left atrium (**Fig. 4**, Video 4); this is often the best view obtained in the patient on mechanical ventilation, as there is no aerated lung to block transmission of ultrasound and the liver serves as an acoustic window. It is the only view that is used for rapid assessment of cardiac function while the pulse is being checked during performance of cardiopulmonary resuscitation.

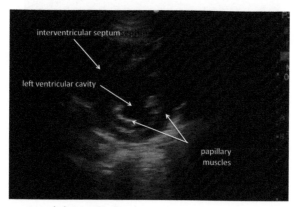

Fig. 2. Normal parasternal short-axis view.

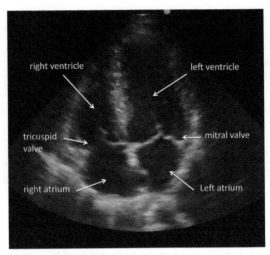

Fig. 3. Normal apical 4-chamber view.

This view allows for assessment of LV/RV size and function, the RV/LV ratio, and for pericardial effusion. Pitfalls of this view include inaccurate assessment of cardiac anatomy and function when the view is off-axis.

Inferior vena cava longitudinal view

From the SCL view, the probe is rotated counterclockwise until the orientation marker is pointed toward the 12 o'clock position (**Fig. 5**, Video 5). The tomographic plane is adjusted by angling the transducer to the left, to visualize the IVC in the longitudinal axis.

This view allows for assessment of preload sensitivity and the presence of pericardial tamponade (the IVC is enlarged with tamponade). Pitfalls of this view include confusing the aorta for the IVC and interpreting respiratory translational artifact as representing respirophasic variation of the IVC.

Clinical Applications of Basic Critical Care Echocardiography

Hemodynamic failure is a common problem in the critically ill patient. In approaching this problem, the intensivist combines the history, physical examination, laboratory

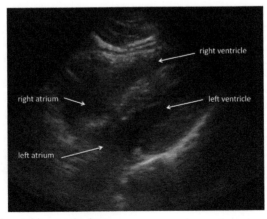

Fig. 4. Normal subcostal long-axis view.

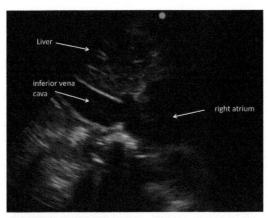

Fig. 5. Inferior vena cava long-axis view.

studies, and standard imaging studies with basic CCE to establish diagnosis and to guide management. The basic CCE examination is not performed in isolation but is combined with the other information to allow the frontline clinician to answer the following questions:

- Is there an imminently life-threatening cause for the hemodynamic failure such as massive valvular failure, pericardial tamponade, acute cor pulmonale caused by a massive pulmonary embolism, or severe hypovolemia with end-systolic efface- ment of the left ventricle?
- What is the category of hemodynamic failure? Is it obstructive, hypovolemic, vas- oplegic, or cardiogenic (valvular or pump failure)?
- What is the appropriate initial management strategy? For example, does the patient need vasopressors, inotropes, fluids, thrombolytics, a mechanical assist device, cardiac surgery, or another intervention?
- What is the response to therapy? For example, is the volume resuscitation adequate? Have the thrombolytics been effective?
- Is there an additional cause for the hemodynamic failure or coexisting condition that will complicate management such as preexisting LV failure, acute cor pulmo- nale with pericardial tamponade, or sepsis with aortic stenosis?
- What are the results of repeated CCE examination during the ICU stay? For example, is there improvement in LV systolic function following treatment of sepsis? Is there improvement of RV systolic function with decreasing levels of positive end-expiratory pressure?
- Is a more comprehensive echocardiography examination required? For example, is there need for measurement of stroke volume (SV), pulmonary pressures, or LA pressure? This type of measurement requires skill in advanced CCE.

Important Elements of the Basic Critical Care Echocardiography Examination

Assessment of preload responsiveness
Respirophasic variation of IVC size predicts fluid responsiveness in the patient with hemodynamic failure. The IVC longitudinal view allows the examiner to measure the size of the IVC during inspiration and expiration. Use of M-mode facilitates the mea- surement, as the caliper function can be used to determine the diameter of the IVC from a frozen image. Respiratory variation of the IVC is a validated method for the

assessment of fluid responsiveness.[6–8] Respiratory variation of greater than 18% (by using [maximum minus minimum]/mean) and 12% (by using [maximum minus minimum]/minimum) identify fluid responsiveness. There are limitations to this technique.

- The patient must be on mechanical ventilatory support and without any spontaneous respiratory effort.
- The degree of IVC variation may vary according to the set tidal volume; larger tidal volumes will result in larger IVC variation.
- Intra-abdominal pressure may influence the degree of IVC variation.
- Respiratory translational artifact may cause movement of the IVC out of the scanning plane, giving the false impression of change in absolute size of the IVC, when the measurement change occurs as an artifact of target movement.
- Whereas a large respirophasic variation of the IVC is readily identified, smaller, but relevant variations are more difficult to measure accurately.

In the spontaneously breathing patient, expert opinion suggests that if the IVC diameter is greater than 2.5 cm, there is a low probability of fluid responsiveness; and if the IVC diameter is less than 1 cm, there is a high probability of fluid responsiveness.[9]

Global left ventricular systolic function

The basic CCE examination allows the intensivist to assess global LV systolic function. The assessment is qualitative, and graded as severely reduced (Video 6), moderately reduced (Video 7), normal (see Video 1), or hyperdynamic (Video 8). Hyperdynamic function is characterized by end-systolic effacement of the LV cavity. Reduced diastolic excursion of the anterior leaflet of the MV is associated with severely decreased LV function. Qualitative assessment of LV function has utility for determination of management strategy for the patient with hemodynamic failure; that is, to guide the use of inotropes, vasopressors, and volume resuscitation. Detailed segmental wall-motion analysis, measurement of SV, and determination of ejection fraction is beyond the scope of basic CCE.

Acute cor pulmonale

Acute cor pulmonale results in characteristic findings with the basic CCE examination.[10] Paradoxic end-systolic movement of the interventricular septum during systole is consistent with RV pressure overload (Video 9), identified in the PSS view and recognized qualitatively as a septal dyskinesia ("septal bounce"). With RV pressure overload, the duration of RV systole is prolonged relative to the left ventricle. For this reason, end-systolic RV pressure is transiently higher than end-systolic LV pressure; so that the interventricular septum is displaced transiently to the left. This phenomenon may be observed with M-mode interrogation. Diastolic overload of the right ventricle results in RV dilatation, identified by end-diastolic size comparison of the right and left ventricles in the AP4 or SCL views (Video 10). Qualitative visual assessment of the ratio is as accurate as quantitative planimetry measurement.[11] An RV:LV ratio of less than 0.6 is normal, between 0.6 and 1 moderate dilatation, and 1 or greater severe RV dilatation. Measurement of RV free wall thickness may be made from the SCL or AP4 views. Normally, RV wall thickness is less than 3 mm. Dilatation of the RV with a normal RV free wall thickness suggests an acute disease process, whereas the finding of increased RV free wall thickness with acute cor pulmonale pattern suggests that the RV has been under longer standing load.

Pericardial tamponade

Pericardial tamponade is always a clinical diagnosis. Echocardiographic features support the diagnosis in the appropriate clinical setting, but cannot be used as the sole means of diagnosis. A pericardial effusion is identified as a relatively hypoechoic space surrounding the heart. On the PSL view, a pericardial effusion is located anterior to the descending thoracic aorta, in contrast to a pleural effusion, which is located posterior to the descending thoracic aorta (Video 11). Pericardial tamponade has characteristic findings with the basic CCE examination (Video 12):

- Dilatation of the IVC without respirophasic size variation
- Swinging of the heart within the pericardial effusion
- Collapse of the right atrium during systole
- Collapse of the right ventricle during diastole
- Accentuated respirophasic variation of RV size

Valve function and pathology

The basic CCE examination may identify major valve abnormalities that are visible on 2-dimensional imaging such as severe aortic stenosis (Video 13), large valvular vegetations (Video 14), or papillary muscle rupture (Video 15). Color Doppler is part of basic CCE, and is used to identify severe valve regurgitation. Although skill at spectral Doppler analysis is not part of basic CCE, proficiency at advanced CCE is required if full evaluation of valve function is required.

Limitations of Basic Critical Care Echocardiography

- As the results of basic CCE have major implications for diagnosis and management, it is required that the intensivist has a high level of skill. Skill at basic CCE may seem, to some trainees, as easy to acquire; this is not the case. The training sequence needs to emphasize skill at image acquisition; multiple studies on normal subjects, followed by patients, are required to reach competence in this key part of basic CCE. High-fidelity TTE and TEE simulators are available that demonstrate pathologic findings; these may facilitate initial training.[12–14] Training includes review of a comprehensive image set that features numerous variations of normal and abnormal findings. The trainee must also master the cognitive base of the field, now widely available in articles, textbooks, and Internet-based resources. To ensure the adequacy of training, formal summative competency-based testing is important at the end of the training period.
- The basic CCE examination is limited in scope. The intensivist performing basic CCE needs know when to call for an advanced level of study.
- It is often difficult to obtain high-quality images in the critically ill patient. At times, the images of both basic and advanced CCE would be considered unacceptable by cardiology standards. Nevertheless, the critical care clinician needs to interpret and apply the results obtained at the bedside, even if they are limited in quality.
- Ideally every basic CCE examination image set should be recorded in a durable and accessible format for later review and comparison, and a formal report should be entered into the patient's medical record. This procedure requires an archiving and communication system that is integrated into the portable ultrasonography machine. This capability is not yet available in most ICUs, with the result that it is difficult to document and store video clips and reports of basic CCE. In the absence of an organized archiving system, in a busy ICU the team performs numerous ultrasonography examinations in rapid sequence. In this scenario, patient care takes precedence over documentation. At a minimum, a short report documenting the findings of the examination is entered in the patient's chart.

Support for Basic Critical Care Echocardiography

To the frontline intensivist, the utility of basic CCE is intuitively obvious. Is there literature to support its clinical utility? Manasia and colleagues[15] report that a goal-directed TTE examination could be performed with a high degree of accuracy, and yielded results that changed therapy in 37% of cases. When combined with other elements of CCUS, Volpicelli and colleagues[16] achieved perfect concordance with final diagnosis of the cause of shock, using an approach that included basic CCE. Laursen and colleagues[17] reported similar results, with focused ultrasonography diagnosing previously missed life-threatening conditions. When combined with other aspects of CCUS, Volpicelli and colleagues[16] required on average 4.9 minutes to perform an ultrasonography examination including basic CCE. Given its ease of use and demonstrated diagnostic utility, the basic CCE examination is a standard part of the evaluation of every patient with hemodynamic failure.

Basic Critical Care Echocardiography and Transesophageal Echocardiography

Although TEE is generally associated with advanced CCE, Benjamin and colleagues[18] reported that a goal-directed TEE examination could be performed by intensivists with limited training, with results that were clinically relevant. The number of views was limited to 4; this gives information similar to that of the basic CCE examination with TTE. Recently, a miniaturized TEE probe has been developed. It is 5.5 mm in diameter and is designed for both oral and nasal insertion. It can be left in place for up to 72 hours; and during this period repeated studies can be performed as guided by clinical need. The device uses a monoplane transducer to obtain 3 views of the heart: the superior vena cava (SVC) transverse view to assess preload sensitivity, the mid-esophageal 4-chamber view to assess RV:LV size ratio, and the transgastric mid-ventricular view to assess LV function and septal kinetics. The device can be used to identify pericardial effusion. It has color Doppler capability, although it lacks spectral Doppler. Several studies have demonstrated the safety, feasibility, and clinical applications of this miniaturized probe.[19] Outcomes studies and direct comparison with TTE have not yet been reported.

Advanced Critical Care Echocardiography: Transthoracic Echocardiography and Transesophageal Echocardiography

Advanced CCE requires competence in all aspects of echocardiography that are standard to cardiology practice, in addition to elements that are particular to critical care medicine.[20–22] Competence in advanced CCE is achieved with a long training period similar in duration to that of the cardiologist who is trained in echocardiography; it includes training in TEE. All intensivists must be competent in basic CCE, whereas only a smaller proportion needs to be proficient in advanced CCE.

Competence in advanced CCE includes proficiency in image acquisition and image interpretation of all standard echocardiography views and Doppler measurements. Use of Doppler permits assessment of hemodynamic function through a variety of pressure and flow measurements, including quantitative measurement of SV, cardiac output, intracardiac pressures, preload sensitivity, and valve function.

THORACIC: PLEURA AND LUNG

Ultrasonographic examination of the lung and pleura is easy to learn and has wide application for the intensivist. Thoracic ultrasonography is superior to standard chest radiography in the ICU, where the supine, rotated, anterior-posterior chest film of variable penetration frequently yields a nonspecific radio-opacity pattern. When compared with computed tomography (CT) of the chest, thoracic ultrasonography is similar in performance for identifying pneumothorax, normal aeration pattern, alveolar-interstitial abnormality, consolidation, and pleural effusion.[23,24] Ultrasonography can largely replace standard chest radiographs in the ICU[25,26] and can greatly reduce the use of chest CT, with concomitant improvement in resource allocation and reduction in radiation exposure.[27] The examination can be performed in a goal-directed fashion and may be repeated as often as required.

Equipment Requirements

The phased-array transducer used for cardiac imaging is effective for lung and pleural ultrasonography. Some machines have a lung preset that automatically optimizes machine settings for lung imaging. If not, the abdominal preset is usually appropriate for thoracic imaging, although the operator may need to make further adjustment. The vascular transducer is used for detailed examination of pleural morphology.

Pleural ultrasonography

Ultrasonography is well suited for the identification of pleural fluid, being as effective as chest CT for this application. The probe is used to examine through adjacent interspaces, and is moved freely over the chest while searching for pleural fluid using a longitudinal scanning plane. By convention, the orientation marker is on the left side of the screen and the probe marker is orientated toward the head of the patient. Unless loculated, pleural fluid assumes a dependent position in the thorax of the supine patient. The detection of smaller effusions requires the scanner to push the probe into the bed mattress with the tomographic plane pointing toward central body mass. Larger effusions may be detected when scanning in the midaxillary line. Pleural fluid is characterized by the following (**Fig. 6**, Video 16).

- Typical anatomic boundaries, which require definitive identification of the diaphragm and subdiaphragmatic organs (liver and spleen, depending on the side), the heart (on the left side), the chest wall, and the surface of the lung.
- Hypoechoic space, which requires definitive identification of a relatively echo-free space that is the pleural effusion, which is surrounded by the typical anatomic boundaries.

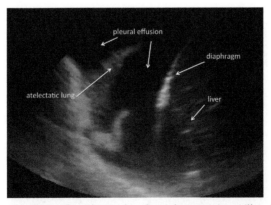

Fig. 6. Pleural effusion. The probe is located in the right posterior axillary line; the anechoic area represents pleural effusion. This image shows an unsafe area for needle insertion, as the lung flap is in the center of the image.

- Dynamic changes, which require definitive identification of changes that are characteristic of a pleural effusion such as diaphragmatic movement, movement of atelectatic lung, and movement of echogenic material within the effusion.

A common application of ultrasonography is to guide safe thoracentesis, which can be accomplished with a high degree of safety in the critically ill on mechanical ventilatory support.[28] Ultrasonography allows identification of a safe trajectory for device insertion that avoids injury to organs surrounding the effusion. This approach requires the operator to make positive identification of the diaphragm (and underlying liver or spleen), the lung, and the heart (for a left-sided effusion). After the procedure, the patient is examined for pneumothorax; presence of lung sliding rules out procedure-related pneumothorax.

Lung ultrasonography

The examination is performed with the phased-array probe using a longitudinal scanning plane with the transducer marker pointed cephalad and the probe held perpendicular to the chest wall. The transducer is moved across the chest wall in a sequence of longitudinal scan lines to examine the lung through adjacent intercostal spaces. This approach allows the examiner to develop a 3-dimensional image of the thorax from multiple 2-dimensional images gathered in an organized scan-line sequence. As with pleural fluid, it is difficult to scan the posterior lung in the supine patient. If necessary, the patient may be positioned in lateral decubitus position.

Important Findings of Lung Ultrasonography

Basic anatomy

With the probe perpendicular to the chest wall and centered on an intercostal space, the examiner will identify the 2 rib shadows on either side of the image. An echogenic line is noted between the rib shadows located 5 mm deep to the periosteum of the adjacent ribs. This feature is the pleural line, and deep to the pleural line is the lung itself (**Fig. 7**, Video 17).

Lung sliding and lung pulse

Lung sliding is identified as respirophasic movement of the pleural line. It indicates that the visceral and parietal pleural surfaces are in apposition to one other, and that there is no pneumothorax at the site of the examination (see Video 17). Multiple sites on the

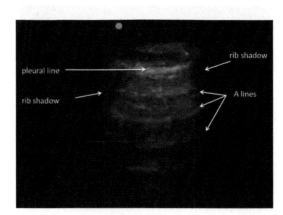

Fig. 7. Longitudinal view through the intercostal space showing, rib shadows, pleural line, and A lines. The presence of A lines suggests a normal aeration pattern in this area.

thorax may be rapidly examined to definitively rule out pneumothorax.[29] Lung pulse is a related finding, whereby cardiophasic movement of the pleura is identified. Lung pulse has the same implication as lung sliding: there is no pneumothorax at the site of the examination (Video 18).[30]

Absence of lung sliding and lung pulse

A pneumothorax results in loss of visceral and parietal pleural apposition, so lung sliding and lung pulse are lost. Other processes can cause loss of lung sliding, such as pleurodesis and severe underlying lung disease (adult respiratory distress syndrome, pneumonia, massive lung bullae), which impede respirophasic movement of the pleural interface. Although the presence of lung sliding rules out pneumothorax in an absolute sense, its absence only suggests pneumothorax. Clinical correlation is required.

Lung point

In the presence of a pneumothorax with partial lung collapse, there will be an interface point between the pneumothorax space and the still aerated but partially collapsed lung. When the vascular transducer is used to scan the lateral intercostal space, it is possible to locate the interface point between the pneumothorax space and the partially deflated lung where intermittent lung sliding is visible. This feature is the lung point, which is diagnostic for the presence of pneumothorax (Video 19).[31]

A lines

On ultrasonography examination, normally aerated lung is characterized by the presence of A lines, defined as 1 or more horizontally oriented lines that are located deep to the pleural line (see Video 17). The first A line is the same distance from the pleural line as is the pleural line from the chest wall. Subsequent A lines, if present, are the same distance from one another. Although a reverberation artifact, A lines are characteristic of normal aerated lung when compared with chest CT.

B lines

The presence of B lines indicates an alveolar or interstitial process at the site of the examination. B lines are strongly correlated with these findings on chest CT.[32] Like any alveolar or interstitial process, they may be focal, multifocal, unilateral, or bilateral depending on the disease involved. B lines have specific characteristics (Video 20). B lines:

- Are vertical in orientation and may occur as 1 or more per field (sometimes termed comet tails or lung rockets)
- Originate at the pleural interface
- Extend to the bottom of the screen
- Efface A lines where the two intersect
- Move in synchrony with lung sliding; however, they are not necessarily mobile, as in the case of B lines in the absence of lung sliding

Other features of B lines include:

- A few B lines may present in normal subjects.
- More than 2 B lines in a single scanning field is abnormal.
- Cardiogenic pulmonary edema results in profuse B lines and a smooth pleural surface.[33]
- Primary lung injury B lines results in focal B lines and an irregular pleural surface.[33]

Consolidation

On lung ultrasonography, consolidation results in tissue-density lung that has the appearance of liver; hence, the term ultrasonographic hepatization of lung has been used to describe this finding (Video 21). Lung consolidation on ultrasonography examination has been strongly correlated with chest CT results.[34] Lung ultrasonography can identify consolidation at the lobar, segmental, subsegmental, and subpleural levels. The finding of consolidation does not imply a specific diagnosis. It may be caused by pneumonia or atelectasis. A pleural effusion causes compressive atelectasis, as does an endobronchial block with resorptive atelectasis. Ultrasonographic air bronchograms are characteristic of pneumonia, whereas their absence suggests endobronchial occlusion with resorptive atelectasis.[35]

Clinical Applications of Lung Ultrasonography

Because lung ultrasonography is superior to standard ICU chest radiography for detection of pneumothorax, normal aeration pattern, alveolar/interstitial abnormality, consolidation, and pleural effusion, it may largely replace standard radiography in the ICU. It also has the advantage of being performed without delay, as often as is required, and with immediate results. Although it is possible to determine the position of central venous lines and gastric tubes with ultrasonography, chest radiography is a more time-efficient way of doing this; hence a check of the device position is still an indication for standard chest radiography in the ICU. Lung ultrasonography has performance characteristics similar to those of chest CT for identification of abnormalities that are of interest to the intensivist, such as listed earlier. Although lung ultrasonography will never entirely replace chest CT, it has the potential to reduce its use. In certain situations, chest CT is superior to lung ultrasonography. Lung lesions that are surrounded by aerated lung and mediastinal structures are not well visualized with thoracic ultrasonography, so chest CT is required to examine these areas. Some specific examples of the use of lung ultrasonography serve to emphasize its broad utility to the intensivist.

- Rapid assessment of acute respiratory failure: Lung ultrasonography can be used in algorithmic fashion to identify the cause of acute respiratory failure.[36]
- Postprocedure evaluation for pneumothorax: Following thoracentesis, central venous access, transthoracic needle aspiration, or transbronchial biopsy, lung ultrasonography can be used to definitively rule out or identify procedure-related pneumothorax[37]; and, in this event, to target an insertion site for pleural drainage. Lung ultrasonography can be used to determine the timing of removal of a pleural drainage device used to treat pneumothorax.[38]
- Resolution of pneumonia: Lung ultrasonography can be used to track the resolution of pneumonia in patients on ventilatory support.[39]
- Identification of lung recruitment: Lung ultrasonography can detect lung recruitment in patients on ventilatory support.[40]
- Estimation of left atrial pressure: Lung ultrasonography can estimate left atrial pressure, and so is useful in determining whether hydrostatic pulmonary edema is present.[41]
- In combination with other elements of CCUS, lung ultrasonography can be used to evaluate hemodynamic and respiratory failure.[16,17]

Limitations of Lung Ultrasonography

The limitations that are relevant to basic CCE hold equally for lung ultrasonography: the need for training, the challenge of the ICU patient who is difficult to image, and the need to know when an alternative imaging technique is required. The problem of documenting the results of the study is a particular challenge with lung ultrasonography. A typical study may have many images, making it difficult to save them in a format that allows direct comparison with previous studies. This problem is compounded by the high volume of studies that may be performed when an ICU team is fully proficient in the technique. Lung ultrasonography is easy to perform and useful for rapid serial assessment, so that a busy ICU team may perform a large number of studies each day. This approach makes documentation of all results a challenging proposition.

GUIDANCE OF VASCULAR ACCESS WITH ULTRASONOGRAPHY
Central Venous Access

The use of ultrasonography to guide central venous access results in increased success and reduced complication rates for access to the internal jugular vein (IJV), subclavian vein (SCV), and common femoral vein (FV). For this reason, it is mandated by the Agency for Healthcare Research and Quality,[42] and is part of routine ICU function. It requires the use of a linear vascular probe (5.0–10.0 MHz) and a purpose-designed sterile probe cover. Real-time imaging of needle insertion is superior to a mark-and-stick approach. The experienced operator will hold the transducer in one hand while inserting the needle with the other. Having a separate operator to hold the probe is both awkward and unnecessary.

Internal Jugular Venous Access

Before applying the sterile field:

- Pneumothorax is ruled out by identification of sliding lung over the anterior thorax bilaterally using the vascular probe.
- Using a transverse scanning plane, both the right and left IJV are examined to look for aberrant anatomy, to identify excessive respirophasic change in vessel diameter, and to perform compression study of both vessels to rule out DVT. With this information, the best side for access is selected.

After applying the sterile field:

- The probe position is adjusted to place the carotid medial to the IJV, to avoid inadvertent carotid puncture.
- The needle is inserted under real-time guidance into the IJV. Most operators use a transverse scanning plane.
- Following wire insertion and needle removal, the IJV is examined in longitudinal scanning plane to document that the wire is inside the IJV lumen before use of the dilator.
- Once the line is secured, pneumothorax is ruled out by identifying sliding lung over the anterior thorax bilaterally using the vascular probe.

Subclavian Venous Access

Before applying the sterile field:

- Pneumothorax is ruled out by identifying sliding lung over the anterior thorax bilaterally using the vascular probe.
- Using a transverse or longitudinal scanning plane, the SCV is scanned to look for aberrant anatomy, to identify excessive respirophasic change in vessel diameter, and to perform compression study to rule out DVT. The SCV may be difficult to compress. Alternative means of distinguishing between the vein and artery

include identifying venous valves or respirophasic variation of the vessel, and by observing augmentation of color Doppler signal with manual compression of the ipsilateral arm.

After applying the sterile field:

- The needle is inserted under real-time guidance in the transverse or longitudinal plane. The insertion site will be more lateral in comparison with the standard landmark technique.
- Following wire insertion and needle removal, the SCV is imaged in longitudinal scanning plane to document that the wire is in the SCV lumen before using the dilator; this may require a supraclavicular window.
- Once the line is secured, pneumothorax is ruled out by identifying sliding lung over the anterior thorax bilaterally using the vascular probe.

Common Femoral Venous Access

Before applying the sterile field:

- Using a transverse scanning plane, both the right and left common FV are imaged to look for aberrant anatomy and to perform compression study of both vessels to rule out DVT. With this information, the best side is selected for access.

After applying the sterile field:

- The probe position is adjusted to identify a trajectory for needle insertion that targets vessel entry into the common FV. Insertion of the needle into the superficial FV risks inadvertent needle entry into the superficial femoral artery, as the artery lies deep to the vein at this anatomic level.
- The needle is inserted under real-time guidance into the common FV. Most operators use a transverse scanning plane.
- Following wire insertion and needle removal, the common FV is imaged in longitudinal scanning plane to document that the wire is in the FV lumen before use of the dilator.

Peripheral Venous Access

Obesity, edema, recreational drug use, or repeated intravenous access requirements make it difficult to insert peripheral intravenous access. Guidance with ultrasonography increases the success rate of peripheral venous access in such patients.[43] The basilic and cephalic veins are often suitable targets. The brachial veins are usually paired and adjacent to the brachial artery, but may also be accessed. Most operators guide needle insertion using a longitudinal scanning plane. Insertion may be guided with a free-hand technique; a needle guide that attaches to the probe may also be used.

Arterial Access

Arterial access, particularly in the radial artery, may present the same challenges as peripheral intravenous access. Guidance with ultrasonography increases the success rate and reduces complications of arterial line insertion.[44]

Vascular Diagnostic: Examination for Deep Venous Thrombosis

Venous thromboembolic disease is often a consideration in the critically ill patient. When it is a possibility, prompt examination for DVT is a key part of the evaluation. Bedside ultrasonography may be performed by the intensivist with a high degree of accuracy.[45] The examination takes a few minutes to perform, can be learned in a short

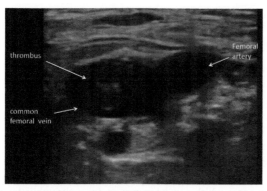

Fig. 8. Thrombus in common femoral vein (FV). Note the echoic defect inside the lumen of the common FV, suggesting the presence of thrombus.

training period, and relies solely on 2-dimensional imaging. Doppler-based measurements are not required.

The examination begins with examination of the target vein using transverse 2-dimensional imaging of the vessel. Normal veins lack internal echoes. A thrombus is seen as a discrete echogenic structure within the venous lumen (**Fig. 8**). If recent, the thrombus may be mobile and relatively hypoechoic. With passage of time, thrombi become gradually more echogenic and less mobile, eventually appearing as an immobile hyperechoic structure that is incorporated into the vessel wall. A thrombus that has formed very recently may be initially anechoic, and can only be identified with compression of the vein by application of pressure with the probe. Normally, veins are fully compressible with light pressure applied with the probe, with the lumen disappearing completely and the venous walls coming into complete contact. A failure to fully compress the venous lumen is evidence for a DVT (Video 22). The amount of pressure applied should be sufficient to deform the adjacent artery.

The examination uses a methodical anatomic approach using the linear vascular probe to obtain a transverse view of the leg veins at defined anatomic levels, as follows:

- Upper common FV (**Fig. 9**, Video 23)
- Common FV at saphenous vein intake level (**Fig. 10**, Video 24)
- Common FV at the bifurcation of the common femoral artery (**Fig. 11**, Video 25)

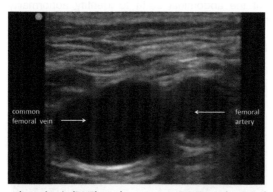

Fig. 9. Deep venous thrombosis (DVT) study, common FV. Note the vein located medially to the artery.

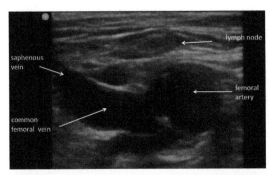

Fig. 10. DVT study, common FV at saphenous vein intake level. Note the lymph node in the upper part of the screen, which can be mistaken for a thrombus by the inexperienced sonographer. Angling of the probe will reveal a spherical structure rather than a vessel.

- Common FV at the deep FV bifurcation level (**Fig. 12**, Video 26)
- Proximal superficial FV level (**Fig. 13**, Video 27)
- Popliteal vein level (at several points along the vein) (**Fig. 14**, Video 28)

At each site, if no thrombus is visible, the examiner proceeds with a venous compression maneuver with the force vector applied perpendicular to the long axis of the vein. The entire length of the superficial FV may be examined; but if the initial sites described here are negative, it is uncommon to find an isolated thrombus in the superficial FV.[46] The axillary, SCV, and IJV may be examined in similar fashion.

Abdominal: Limited Examination

The ACCP/SRLF Statement on Competence describes that competence in a limited abdominal ultrasonography examination is sufficient for the frontline intensivist. Competence in all aspects of abdominal ultrasonography is neither necessary nor feasible, given the complexity of the field. A key element of competence in the limited abdominal examination is that the intensivist knows when to call for a higher-level scanner. Competence in the limited examination includes the following elements.

- Identification of intra-abdominal fluid and determination of a safe trajectory for needle insertion required for paracentesis
- Assessment of the urinary tract (kidney and bladder) to identify abnormality, such as bladder distension, hydronephrosis, and kidney stones
- Assessment of the abdominal aorta to identify abnormality, such as aortic dissection or aneurysm

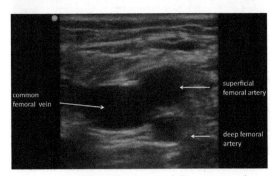

Fig. 11. DVT study, common FV at the bifurcation of the common femoral artery.

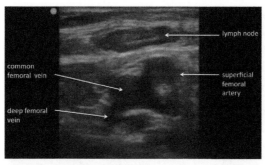

Fig. 12. DVT study, common FV at the deep FV bifurcation level. Note again the presence of a lymph node in the upper part of the screen.

The focused assessment with sonography for trauma (FAST) examination is a standard part of the evaluation of the patient who may have traumatic internal injuries resulting in intra-abdominal bleeding. The finding of intra-abdominal fluid in the trauma patient is strong evidence of visceral injury resulting in bleeding, and is used to guide management strategy. Depending on the particular algorithm used, this may indicate immediate surgical intervention if the patient is unstable. If the patient is stable, it may require further imaging with abdominal CT. If the initial FAST is negative for fluid, it may be repeated at short intervals given that the examination is so easy to perform. Accumulation of fluid following an initially negative result alerts the intensivist to the possibility of ongoing intra-abdominal bleeding.

The FAST examination is performed with the patient in the supine position, and requires 3 standard views[47]:

- On the right side, the probe is placed in the 10th or 11th intercostal space in the posterior axillary line with the indicator pointed cephalad to achieve a coronal scanning plane. The hepatorenal space is examined for fluid. Fluid may also be observed around the liver (**Fig. 15**, Video 29).
- The probe is placed in the suprapubic area with the indicator pointed toward the right to achieve a transverse scanning plane. The transducer is angled so as to orientate the tomographic scanning plane for examination into the pelvis for fluid (**Fig. 16**, Video 30).

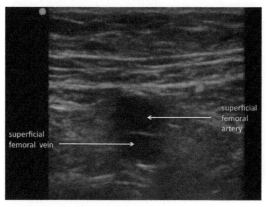

Fig. 13. DVT study, proximal superficial FV level.

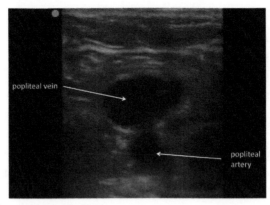

Fig. 14. DVT study, popliteal vein level.

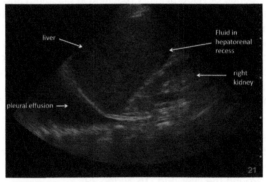

Fig. 15. Intra-abdominal fluid study, right costophrenic angle. There is fluid within the hepatorenal space, with coexisting pleural effusion.

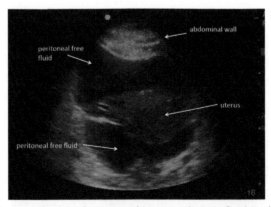

Fig. 16. Intra-abdominal fluid study, suprapubic area. There is fluid in the pelvis with the uterus within the fluid collection.

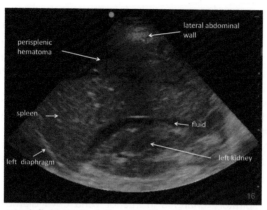

Fig. 17. Intra-abdominal fluid study, left costophrenic angle. There is fluid between the spleen and kidney, and a perisplenic hematoma.

- On the left side, the probe is placed in a position analogous to that on the right side, although the scanning plane may have to be more posterior than on the right side. The perisplenic area is examined for fluid (**Fig. 17**, Video 31).

The FAST examination is frequently combined with other views that are useful for rapid evaluation of the trauma patient. For example, the subcostal cardiac view is performed to evaluate for pericardial effusion, and bilateral examination of the thorax is indicated to evaluate for pneumothorax and hemothorax.

The FAST examination is specific for the management of the trauma patient. In the medical patient, identification of intra-abdominal fluid does not necessarily have the same implications that it has in the trauma patient. Instead, the intensivist considers the etiology of the fluid and whether there is a safe site in which to perform paracentesis. Often the fluid is anechoic, which is characteristic of transudative ascites. Echogenic material and septations are associated with complex ascites. Ultrasonography has utility in guiding paracentesis, as it allows identification of a safe trajectory for needle insertion that avoids injury to organs surrounding the ascites. This approach requires the operator to make positive identification of the diaphragm, intestine, liver, spleen, and bladder. An occasional complication of paracentesis is laceration of an aberrant inferior epigastric artery. Examination of the planned needle trajectory with the vascular probe using color Doppler has been proposed to reduce the risk of this uncommon complication.[48]

SUMMARY

CCUS is a useful skill for the intensivist. Competence in CCUS requires mastery of basic CCE, thoracic, vascular access, vascular diagnostic, and abdominal screening ultrasonography.

SUPPLEMENTARY DATA

Supplementary data related to this article can be found online at http://dx.doi.org/10.1016/j.ccc.2014.08.003.

REFERENCES

1. Mayo PH, Beaulieu Y, Doelken P, et al. American College of Chest Physicians/ Société de Réanimation de Langue Française statement on competence in critical care ultrasonography. Chest 2009;135:1050–60.

2. Cholley BP, Mayo PH, Poelaert J, et al. International expert statement on training standards for critical care ultrasonography. Intensive Care Med 2011;37:1077–83.

3. Accreditation Council for Graduate Medical Education. ACGME program requirements for graduate medical education in critical care medicine. Available at: https://www.acgme.org/acgmeweb/Portals/0/PFAssets/2013-PR-FAQ-PIF/142_critical_care_int_med_07132013.pdf. Accessed September 26, 2014.

4. Vieillard-Baron A, Mayo PH, Vignon P, et al. International consensus statement on training standards for advanced critical care echocardiography. Intensive Care Med 2014;40(5):654–66.

5. Labovitz AJ, Noble VE, Bierig M, et al. Focused cardiac ultrasound in the emergent setting: a consensus statement of the American Society of Echocardiography and American College of Emergency Physicians. J Am Soc Echocardiogr 2010;23:1225–30.

6. Barbier C. Respiratory changes in inferior vena cava diameter are helpful in predicting fluid responsiveness in ventilated septic patients. Intensive Care Med 2004;30:1740–6.

7. Feissel M. The respiratory variation in the inferior vena cava diameter as a guide to fluid therapy. Intensive Care Med 2004;30:1834–7.

8. Moretti R. Inferior vena cava distensibility as a predictor of fluid responsiveness in patients with subarachnoid hemorrhage. Neurocrit Care 2010;13:3–9.

9. Schmidt G, Koenig S, Mayo PH. Shock: ultrasound to guide diagnosis and therapy. Chest 2012;142:1042–8.

10. Kaplan A. Echocardiographic diagnosis and monitoring of right ventricular function. In: Levitov A, Mayo PH, Slonim AD, editors. Critical care ultrasonography. New York: McGraw Hill; 2009. p. 125–34.

11. Vieillard-Baron A, Charron C, Chergui K, et al. Bedside echocardiographic evaluation of hemodynamics in sepsis: is a qualitative evaluation sufficient? Intensive Care Med 2006;32:1547–52.

12. Dorfling J, Hatton KW, Hassan ZU. Integrating echocardiography into human patient simulator training of anesthesiology residents using a severe pulmonary embolism scenario. Simul Healthc 2006;1:79–83.

13. Platts DG, Humphries J, Burstow DJ, et al. The use of computerised simulators for training of transthoracic and transesophageal echocardiography. The future of echocardiography training? Heart Lung Circ 2012;21:267–74.

14. Neelankavil J, Howard-Quijano K, Hsieh TC, et al. Transthoracic echocardiography simulation is an efficient method to train anesthesiologists in basic transthoracic echocardiography skills. Anesth Analg 2012;115:1042–51.

15. Manasia AR, Nagaraj HM, Kodali RB, et al. Feasibility and potential clinical utility of goal-directed transthoracic echocardiography performed by noncardiologist intensivists using a small hand-carried device (SonoHeart) in critically ill patients. J Cardiothorac Vasc Anesth 2005;19:155–9.

16. Volpicelli G, Lamort A, Tullio M, et al. Point-of-care multi-organ ultrasonography for the evaluation of undifferentiated hypotension in the emergency department. Intensive Care Med 2013;39:1290–8.

17. Laursen CB, Sloth E, Lambrechtsen J, et al. Focused sonography of the heart, lungs, and deep veins identifies missed life-threatening conditions in admitted patients with acute respiratory symptoms. Chest 2013;144:1868–75.

18. Benjamin E, Griffin K, Leibowitz AB, et al. Goal-directed transesophageal echocardiography performed by intensivists to assess left ventricular function: comparison with pulmonary artery catheterization. J Cardiothorac Vasc Anesth 1998;12:10–5.

19. Vieillard-Baron A, Slama M, Mayo P, et al. A pilot study on safety and clinical utility of a single-use 72-hour indwelling transesophageal echocardiography probe. Intensive Care Med 2012;39:629–35.
20. De Backer D, Cholley BP, Slama M, et al. Hemodynamic monitoring using echocardiography in the critically ill. Berlin Heidelberg: Springer; 2011.
21. Narasimhan M, Koenig SJ, Mayo PH. Advanced echocardiography for the critical care physician: part 1. Chest 2014;145:129–34.
22. Narasimhan M, Koenig SJ, Mayo PH. Advanced echocardiography for the critical care physician: part 2. Chest 2014;145:135–42.
23. Lichtenstein D, Goldstein I, Mourgeon E, et al. Comparative diagnostic performances of auscultation, chest radiography, and lung ultrasonography in acute respiratory distress syndrome. Anesthesiology 2004;100:9–15.
24. Xirouchaki N, Magkanas E, Vaporidi K, et al. Lung ultrasound in critically ill patients: comparison with bedside chest radiography. Intensive Care Med 2011;37:1488–93.
25. Zanobetti M, Poggioni C, Pini R. Can chest ultrasonography replace standard chest radiography for evaluation of acute dyspnea in the ED? Chest 2011;139: 1140–7.
26. Ioos V, Galbois A, Chalumeau-Lemoine L, et al. An integrated approach for prescribing fewer chest x-rays in the ICU. Ann Intensive Care 2011;1:4.
27. Brenner DJ, Hall EJ. Computed tomography—an increasing source of radiation exposure. N Engl J Med 2007;357:2277–84.
28. Mayo PH, Goltz HR, Tafreshi M, et al. Safety of ultrasound-guided thoracentesis in patients receiving mechanical ventilation. Chest 2004;125:1059–62.
29. Lichtenstein DA, Menu Y. A bedside ultrasound sign ruling out pneumothorax in the critically ill. Lung sliding. Chest 1995;108:1345–8.
30. Lichtenstein DA, Lascols N, Prin S, et al. The "lung pulse": an early ultrasound sign of complete atelectasis. Intensive Care Med 2003;29:2187–92.
31. Lichtenstein D, Mezière G, Biderman P, et al. The "lung point": an ultrasound sign specific to pneumothorax. Intensive Care Med 2000;26:1434–40.
32. Lichtenstein D, Mézière G, Biderman P, et al. The comet-tail artifact. An ultrasound sign of alveolar-interstitial syndrome. Am J Respir Crit Care Med 1997; 156:1640–6.
33. Copetti R, Soldati G, Copetti P. Chest sonography: a useful tool to differentiate acute cardiogenic pulmonary edema from acute respiratory distress syndrome. Cardiovasc Ultrasound 2008;6:1–10.
34. Lichtenstein DA, Lascols N, Mezière G, et al. Ultra-sound diagnosis of alveolar consolidation in the critically ill. Intensive Care Med 2004;30:276–81.
35. Lichtenstein D, Mezière G, Seitz J. The dynamic air bronchogram. A lung ultrasound sign of alveolar consolidation ruling out atelectasis. Chest 2009;135:1421–5.
36. Lichtenstein DA, Meziere GA. Relevance of lung ultrasound in the diagnosis of acute respiratory failure: the BLUE protocol. Chest 2008;134:117–25.
37. Kreuter M, Eberhardt R, Wenz H, et al. Diagnostic value of transthoracic ultrasound compared to chest radiography in the detection of a post-interventional pneumothorax. Ultraschall Med 2011;32(Suppl 2):E20–3.
38. Galbois A, Ait-Oufella H, Baudel JL, et al. Pleural ultrasound compared with chest radiographic detection of pneumothorax resolution after drainage. Chest 2010; 138:648–55.
39. Bouhemad B, Liu ZH, Arbelot C, et al. Ultrasound assessment of antibiotic-induced pulmonary reaeration in ventilator-associated pneumonia. Crit Care Med 2010;38:84–92.

40. Bouhemad B, Bresson H, Le-Guen M, et al. Bedside ultrasound assessment of positive end-expiratory pressure-induced lung recruitment. Am J Respir Crit Care Med 2011;183:341–7.
41. Lichtenstein DA, Mezière GA, Lagoueyte JF, et al. A-lines and B-lines: lung ultrasound as a bedside tool for predicting pulmonary artery occlusion pressure in the critically ill. Chest 2009;136:1014–20.
42. Rothschild JM. Ultrasound guidance of central vein catheterization: Making healthcare safer: a critical analysis of patient safety practices. Available at: http://archive.ahrq.gov/clinic/ptsafety/chap21.htm. Accessed September 26, 2014.
43. Heinrichs J, Fritze Z, Vandermeer B, et al. Ultrasonographically guided peripheral intravenous cannulation of children and adults: a systematic review and meta-analysis. Ann Emerg Med 2013;61:444–54.
44. Shiloh AL, Savel RH, Paulin LM, et al. Ultrasound-guided catheterization of the radial artery: a systematic review and meta-analysis of randomized controlled trials. Chest 2011;139:524–9.
45. Kory PD, Pellecchia CM, Shiloh A, et al. Accuracy of ultrasonography performed by critical care physicians for the diagnosis of deep venous thrombosis Koenig. Chest 2011;139:538–42.
46. Cogo A, Lensing AW, Prandoni P, et al. Distribution of thrombosis in patients with symptomatic deep vein thrombosis implications for simplifying the diagnostic process with compression ultrasound. Arch Intern Med 1993;153:2777–80.
47. Ma OJ, Kefer MP, Mateer JR, et al. Evaluation of hemoperitoneum using a single-versus multiple-view ultrasonographic examination. Acad Emerg Med 1995;2:581–6.
48. Sekiguchi H, Suzuki J, Daniels CE. Making paracentesis safer: a proposal for the use of bedside abdominal and vascular ultrasonography to prevent a fatal complication. Chest 2013;143:1136–9.

Invasive Hemodynamic Monitoring

Sheldon Magder, MD

KEYWORDS

- Cardiac output • Central venous pressure • Pulmonary artery catheter
- Pulmonary artery occlusion pressure • Pulmonary pressure

KEY POINTS

- Proper use of invasive monitoring must begin with careful attention to the details of making the measurements and making the measurements safely.
- A useful start in managing hypotension is to consider whether the problem is a cardiac output problem or a systemic vascular resistance problem.
- If the cardiac output is the primary problem, the next question is whether this is due to a cardiac function problem or return problem (venous return).
- Measurements of cardiac output and central venous pressure are central to separating these possibilities.
- Trends in cardiac output and central venous pressure are more useful than static measures.
- Pressure tracings can provide diagnostic information beyond the simple hemodynamic measures, including indications of pulmonary function.

INTRODUCTION

The use of invasive hemodynamic monitoring has decreased significantly over the past 2 decades. An important likely factor is failure to find an effect on outcome in an evidence-based medicine driven approach to patient management.[1] However, lack of evidence of benefit does not mean that there is no benefit. Studies on the use of pulmonary artery catheters (PACs) have been limited by lack of algorithms that can show their usefulness, lack of precision in making the measurements, and lack of physiologic rationale of what actually can be fixed based on the information obtained.[2–5] Invasive monitoring also requires a greater skill set on the part of the practitioner, yet studies have shown a striking lack of knowledge of the measurements obtained with the PAC.[6,7] Another issue is the risks associated with insertion of the

Disclosure: None.
Department of Critical Care, Royal Victoria Hospital, McGill University Health Centre, 687 Pine Avenue West, Montreal, Quebec H3A 1A1, Canada
E-mail address: sheldon.magder@muhc.mcgill.ca

Crit Care Clin 31 (2015) 67–87
http://dx.doi.org/10.1016/j.ccc.2014.08.004
0749-0704/15/$ – see front matter
criticalcare.theclinics.com

catheter. However, a major component of such risks is the insertion of a central venous line, which needs to be inserted anyway in most critically ill patients to allow infusion of vasoactive drugs. Furthermore, less invasive devices are not necessarily noninvasive and carry risks of their own, including cannulation of brachial or femoral arteries, which are more invasive than the simple insertion of radial artery catheters. In general, the less invasive the device the less accurate, precise, and reliable it is. Less invasive devices cost more than the simple PAC and the information they give also is more limited. Although the complexity of clinical problems makes it difficult to rigorously establish a role for PACs in randomized trials, the author's sense is that there will likely remain a place for their use in complex patients who are difficult to manage. However, use of PACs requires knowledge of how to use them properly. This article begins with a short review of the basic physiology that determines cardiac output and blood pressure, thus to understand how the measurements obtained can be used for both diagnosis and direct management. Data from a PAC only can be useful if properly measured, so the basics of making such measurements are reviewed. Use of the PAC in making a diagnosis and for management is addressed; these are not the same, and the emphasis is on the use of a responsive approach to management. Finally, the author explores uses of the PAC that are not indications by themselves for placing the catheter, but can provide useful information when a PAC is in place.

Purpose of the Circulation

The primary purpose of the circulation is to deliver the appropriate amount of oxygen and nutrients to the tissues to meet their needs and to remove wastes. The delivery of oxygen (Do_2) is determined by the product of cardiac output (Q), hemoglobin concentration ([Hgb]), and the saturation of hemoglobin, which in turn is determined by the partial pressure of oxygen (Po_2) and a constant (K) that gives the O_2-carrying capacity of hemoglobin:

$$Do_2 = Q \times [Hgb] \times O_2 \text{ saturation} \times K$$

Values for K used in the literature vary from 1.34 to 1.39. Isolated pure hemoglobin carries 1.39 mL O_2 per gram, but blood also has methemoglobin and carboxyhemoglobin so that lower empiric values for K are used for determining the oxygen content in blood. This simple equation indicates that only 3 variables can increase or decrease Do_2. The range of manipulation of hemoglobin is usually not large, and that of saturation even less. For example, an increase in arterial O_2 saturation from 85% to 100% only increases Do_2 by 18% and increases [Hgb] from 90 to 100 g/L by 11%. It should thus be evident that cardiac output is the primary variable that can be manipulated for making major changes in Do_2.

Regulation of Cardiac Output

Cardiac output is determined by the interaction of cardiac function and a function that defines the return of blood to the heart (venous return function) (**Fig. 1**).[8,9] A key implication of this statement is that the heart only can pump out what comes back to it. In turn, this is primarily determined by the properties of venous drainage back to the heart because almost 70% of blood volume is in small systemic veins and venules.[10] By stretching the small veins and venules, this volume creates an elastic recoil pressure that drives flow back to the heart through the small resistance that separates the venous reservoir from the right heart.[8,9] In this analysis arterial blood pressure does not have a significant impact on the return of blood to the heart, for it is the volume

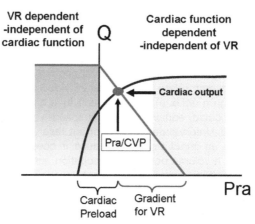

Fig. 1. Cardiac output and right atrial pressure (Pra) are determined by the interaction of cardiac function and return function (venous return [VR]). On the flat part of the cardiac function curve, cardiac output is independent of VR. On the flat part of the VR curve, cardiac output is independent of cardiac function. CVP, central venous pressure.

per minute filling the veins and venules rather than the arterial inflow pressure that determines venous emptying. Changes in cardiac function increase or decrease cardiac output by regulating right atrial pressure and allowing more or less blood to return per beat. When cardiac function increases, the same cardiac output can occur with a lower right atrial pressure. This "permissive" action increases the gradient for venous return, and allows more blood to come back to the heart and to be pumped out. Cardiac function is increased by an increase in heart rate, increase in contractility, or decrease in afterload, which is essentially the arterial pressure in the main pulmonary artery and aorta. The cardiac function curve is also limited by the maximum end-diastolic volume.[11] In the right heart this occurs in most people at a right atrial pressure of 10 to 12 mm Hg (when measured by a fluid-filled pressure transducer whose zero pressure reference is made 5 cm vertical distance below the sternal angle),[12] and once this limit is reached, further increases in preload do not increase cardiac output and an increase in cardiac function is required to increase cardiac output. The maximum potential for increases in cardiac function to increase cardiac output occurs when the right atrial pressure is at or below atmospheric pressure when breathing is spontaneous. However, during positive pressure ventilation, pleural pressure is greater than atmospheric pressure so that right atrial pressure rises with pleural pressure and decreases the pressure gradient for venous return. The range of right ventricular preloads that can alter cardiac output, estimated as right atrial pressure, is small, ranging from 0 to 10 mm Hg in most people. Thus, large increases in cardiac output also require adjustments in the venous return function that are discussed next.

The determinants of venous return are the stressed vascular volume, the resistance draining the venous compartment (venous resistance), the compliance of veins and venules, and the outflow pressure of the venous system, which is the right atrial pressure.[9] Stressed volume refers to the volume that actually stretches the elastic walls of blood vessels. Under resting conditions only about 30% of blood volume, or approximately 1.3 to 1.4 L, actually does this.[13] The rest of the volume just fills out the vessels and is "unstressed." Neural-humeral mechanisms can tighten vessels and convert unstressed volume into stressed volume. In someone who is volume replete, approximately 10 mL/kg to even as much as 18 mL/kg of unstressed volume can be recruited into stressed volume by what is termed a decrease in capacitance.[10,14] A decrease in capacitance increases the upstream venous pressure and thereby increases venous return. To understand the magnitude of the effect of a decrease in capacitance on the circulation, 10 mL/kg in a 70-kg person would increase stressed volume by more than 50% and could increase cardiac output by almost 5 L/min if the heart was able to accommodate the increase in venous return. This recruitment of volume occurs through a reflex mechanism, and thus occurs in seconds. An increase in capacitance could equally reduce stressed volume very rapidly and decrease cardiac output. Unfortunately the important reserve of unstressed volume cannot be measured in an intact person, because it does not produce anything measurable. The use of a volume bolus in resuscitation acts in the same way as a decrease in capacitance. It increases the upstream venous pressure and thereby increases venous return. However, only volume that remains in the vasculature can serve this function. Increasing stressed volume increases capillary pressure, which increases capillary filtration. The net increase in intravascular volume is thus reduced, as is the potential of increasing stressed volume to maintain the transient increase in the venous return function.

A decrease in venous resistance also increases venous return, and does so without increasing upstream venous pressure. This mechanism is important for production of the high cardiac output that occurs during aerobic exercise,[15] but also likely contributes to the increase in cardiac output in septic shock.[16]

An increase in venous return function only can increase cardiac output if the heart is functioning on the ascending part of the cardiac function curve; this, too, greatly limits how much can be achieved by giving fluids. When the right heart becomes volume limited, only an increase in cardiac function can result in an increase in cardiac output (see **Fig. 1**).

Safety Issues

Attention to safety can reduce potential harm with the use of a PAC. This article deals with some important specific issues. Insertion of central venous lines and PACs needs to be done under sterile conditions[17,18] including the use of gown, gloves, face-mask, and sterile drapery that completely covers the patient. The balloon on the catheter should be inflated ex vivo before insertion to ensure that it is intact and that it does not expand asymmetrically. The displayed distal tip vascular pressure and the associated electrocardiogram (ECG) rhythm must be carefully watched on the bedside monitor for arrhythmias and changes in vascular pressure while the catheter is floated through the heart with the balloon inflated, along with immediate awareness of the amount of catheter inserted in centimeters. Because the wave patterns indicate where the end of the catheter is located, it is essential to know what these waveforms should look like as the tip passes from the vena cava through the right heart and into the pulmonary artery (**Figs. 2–4**). Before starting PAC insertion, it is important to ensure that the transducer sensing this pressure is leveled properly so that pressure is measured relative to a standard reference level. If an arrhythmia occurs during placement, and the catheter has to be rapidly pulled out, this may be the only measurement obtained. On a practical level, gently shaking the catheter and noting the paired sinusoidal pressure response on the monitor is useful for validating that the pressure is being seen on the monitor and that the gain on the monitor is appropriately set for the patient's expected hemodynamic values. PAC insertion is usually done through an internal jugular access point, using a specially modified catheter sheath that can continually infuse fluids through a side port while allowing PAC insertion through the central lumen. On insertion, the pressure waveform

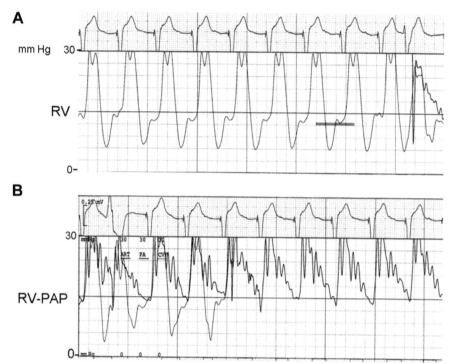

Fig. 2. Right ventricular (RV) (*A*) and pulmonary artery tracing (*B*) in a spontaneously breathing subject. The rhythm, top row of *A* and *B*, is sinus with atrial sensing ventricular pacing. The horizontal line in *A* indicates the preload of the right heart. The first 4 beats of *B* show both RV and pulmonary artery pressure (PAP) tracings and then only PAP. The second beat is a ventricular ectopic.

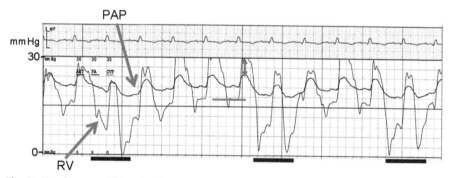

Fig. 3. Simultaneous RV and pulmonary artery tracings obtained by advancing the PAC so that the proximal port is in the right ventricle. The RV diastolic pressure is almost 18 mm Hg (*horizontal line*) and has a marked respiratory variation. There is a pressure gradient between the peak systolic RV pressure and PAP pressure (*shown by double arrow*), which is especially apparent during expiration. The subject had a heart transplant, and the gradient is likely because the pulmonary artery anastomosis was too tight.

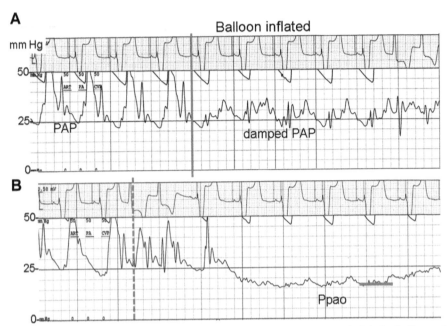

Fig. 4. Pulmonary artery and pulmonary artery occlusion pressure (Ppao). (*A*) The balloon of the PAC is inflated and the wave may appear to be a Ppao, but is actually a "damped" PAP. (*B*) The trace again starts with PAP, and the balloon is inflated at the vertical dotted line; the PAP dampens in the next 3 beats and then finally occludes the pulmonary artery and gives the true Ppao. The horizontal line shows where to measure Ppao (16 mm Hg).

changes into a low-pressure but spiked waveform signal on entering the right atrium. At around 30 cm in average-sized adults, the tricuspid valve is passed and a right ventricular pressure tracing is seen. If the right ventricular pressure recording does not occur following a right atrial pressure recording, the catheter may be coiled in the right atrium or may have passed down the inferior vena cava. Extreme care during insertion must be taken to prevent excess insertion for coiling of the catheter can occur, with the risk of creating a knot in the catheter that makes removal difficult. The pulmonary artery is usually reached by 40 to 45 cm and the pulmonary artery becomes occluded by the balloon (pulmonary artery occlusion pressure [Ppao]) from around 45 to 55 cm, although this can occasionally be farther if the right ventricle is very large. Insertion of the PAC much beyond these length limits again increases the risk of tangling the catheter. Once properly placed and noting that occlusion can be performed, a chest radiograph needs to be performed. A useful practice is to allow the tip of the catheter to remain within the mediastinal shadow because of the risk of pulmonary artery rupture if the PAC tip is farther out and continually striking the pulmonary arterial wall with each contraction. Occasionally this may mean that an occlusion pressure cannot be obtained in this new position. If so, selective readvancement of the PAC during times when Ppao measures are needed is a reasonable option, returning the PAC back to its withdrawn position afterward. Because the Ppao is more useful for diagnostic purposes than to titrate therapy, its measurement does not need to be made often. Furthermore, Ppao can be related to the pulmonary diastolic pressure, and trends in the pulmonary diastolic pressure can then be followed unless a more precise Ppao is needed. If the PAC is inserted beyond

55 cm, one should be especially careful to ensure that there is not a double loop in the right atrium by looking at the chest radiograph. Finally, the PAC balloon should never be left inflated if not being used for balloon inflation PAC insertion or for the measurements of Ppao.

PRESSURE MEASUREMENTS

Measurement of pressure requires care because there are many sources of error and artifacts.[19] Three things always must be considered when measuring pressure: zeroing, leveling, and calibration. Pressure-sensing catheters are all filled with fluid. PACs are fluid-filled catheters with multiple lumens, all attached to transducers. The pressure transducers contain a conductive material surrounded by a series of resistors that ensures constant voltage across the material. This electrical circuit is called a Wheatstone bridge. A change in pressure on the surface of the material changes its electrical resistance, producing a measurable change in current. Application of known forces to the device are used to "calibrate" the relation between the current change in external pressure, such that the force of the vascular pressure applied on the surface of the sensor causes a change in current, which is linearly related to the change in pressure. This measurement setup introduces 3 potential errors, the first related to the background pressure, another to gain, and the final one to the force of gravity and the weight of the fluid in the system. We are surrounded by atmospheric pressure, which is not zero but 760 mm Hg and, thus, almost 8 times the magnitude of arterial pressure and close to almost 1000 times the central venous pressure in the upright position. However, because the outside perimeter of the body senses this atmospheric pressure equally, atmospheric pressure can be used as a reference background pressure; this is dealt with by opening the membrane of the transducer to the surrounding air and calling this value zero. Positive or negative pressure measurements then are deviations from this reference value. Unless one is in the middle of a hurricane, atmospheric pressure changes slowly and by small amounts, so that once the device is zeroed changes in atmospheric pressure do not affect short-term values. The electronics of modern devices also do not have a "drift" in the zero measurement that was common in older devices, although such electromechanical zero-balance drift still can occur if there is an electronic malfunction. Drift is easily identified by opening the transducer to air and observing if the value is or is not still zero. Once the sensor is zeroed, a fixed known pressure signal is applied to the pressure transducer and the observed increase in sensed pressure noted. Usually an electronic validated mock signal of 100 mm Hg is applied to the transducer. However, one could just as easily apply a column of water or mercury to the tip of the transducer and note the gain. Some monitors allow the gain of the system to be changed either up or down, so that the external pressure signal causes the defined reported pressure to change. Many modern systems do not allow this calibration to be done because the pressure transducers are calibrated by the factory. Nevertheless, a good monitoring service, such as an intensive care unit or operating room, should periodically test the accuracy of the calibration of their pressure transducers using external pressure-generating devices (eg, blood pressure cuff).

The third issue in measuring vascular pressure is leveling, and is also the most troublesome. When measuring pressure in fluid-filled systems, the fluid within the catheter lumen has a weight resulting from the force of gravity, and this force is proportional to the height of the fluid column and its density. The density of water is 1, and the density of blood is close to that value. The effect of the gravitational force can be large. In the upright posture, gravity adds a pressure to the veins in the feet that is almost equal to mean arterial pressure.[20] The key point is that measurements in fluid systems are relative to where the properly zeroed transducer is placed. This decision is an arbitrary one, but in controlled physiologic studies the consensus is that this level should be at the mid-point of the right atrium, because at this location blood comes back to the heart before being ejected again.[21] This level can be approximated in an intact person by first identifying the sternal angle, which is where the second rib joins the sternum, then using a leveling device and dropping a line to 5 cm vertical distance from this point. This position is a good approximation in a person lying flat or sitting up to a 60° angle, because the right atrium is a relatively round structure and just below the sternum. There is some variation with body size and heart size, but at least always using a fixed point allows trends in values to be tracked whether the person is lying flat or is partially upright. More commonly the level is taken at the mid-axillary or mid-thoracic line in the fourth intercostal space. The advantage of this approach is that it does not require a leveling device. However, that may also be its disadvantage because the choice of this position is not done as carefully, resulting in greater variation among personnel. Measurement from the mid-axillary line also should be made with the patient supine, as the position of the mid-point of the right atrium moves relative to the mid-axillary line with changes in posture. In some situations, for example, in the operating room, one does not have a choice because the sternal angle and/or part of the surgical field is covered. On average, the mid-thoracic measurement is 3 mm Hg greater than the sternal angle–based approach, but the exact difference depends on chest size.[12] In this article the sternal angle–based reference is used for measurements.

The major energy producing the pressures that are important in hemodynamics is elastic energy. This force stretches the walls of the cardiac chambers and vessels, and determines filtration across capillary membranes. Moreover it creates a pressure difference between the inside and outside elastic structures, called transmural pressure. For structures that are not in the chest the pressure outside their walls is atmospheric pressure, which is zero (see earlier discussion). Thus the measured pressure with a transducer zeroed to atmosphere is the transmural pressure (inside pressure minus zero). However, if the surrounding pressure is greater than zero then actual pressure distending a vessel is less than intramural pressure alone. For example, under conditions of increased intracranial pressure following head trauma, cerebral perfusion pressure is mean arterial pressure minus intracranial pressure, not mean arterial pressure alone. Similarly, if intra-abdominal hypertension develops, intra-abdominal organ perfusion pressure will be mean arterial pressure minus intra-abdominal pressure. The same is true for structures inside the chest, as they are surrounded by pleural pressure, and pleural pressure can vary widely during breathing and with the application of positive end-expiratory pressure.[19,22] At resting end-expiration, referred to as functional residual capacity, the recoil of the lung inward and the chest wall outward produces a pleural pressure that is negative relative to atmospheric pressure. During spontaneous breaths pleural pressure falls further relative to atmospheric pressure owing to active chest wall expansion by the respiratory muscles, and during positive pressure breaths and the application of positive end-expiratory pressure (PEEP), pleural pressure increases relative to atmospheric pressure as a function of both lung and chest wall compliance. Thus, vascular pressures measured with standard pressure transducers no longer represent intrathoracic vascular transmural pressure. There is no simple way to eliminate this problem, but it can be minimized by always making intrathoracic vascular pressure measurements at the end of expiration (which is the same as pre-inspiration), because at this point pleural pressure is closest to atmospheric pressure. However, if a patient is receiving high levels of PEEP, end-expiratory pleural pressure may be elevated and the vascular pressure value seen on the monitor will overestimate the transmural pressure. In normal subjects, with normal lung and chest wall compliance, a little less than half of the airway pressure is transmitted to the pleural space, meaning that with a PEEP of 5 cm H_2O less than 2 mm Hg is transmitted to the pleural space. The stiffer the lung, the less the transmission of airway pressure to the pleural space, so that even patients with high values of PEEP may not have large increases in pleural pressure if they also have acute lung injury. Unfortunately, there is no simple formula that is valid for all patients. It also is not valid to remove the PEEP to measure these intrathoracic vascular pressures because removing PEEP also changes the hemodynamics. It is possible to examine the effect of PEEP on the Ppao by rapidly removing the PEEP and observing the nadir of the decrease in the Ppao after 2 to 3 seconds,[23] but this cannot be used for the central venous pressure (CVP)/right atrial pressure because of the rapid changes in right heart filling along with changes in intrathoracic pressure. One method to estimate transmural Ppao is to compare the change in end-expiratory airway plateau pressure with PEEP as the delta airway pressure to the change in pulmonary artery diastolic pressure from end-expiration to end-inspiration. Because pulmonary arterial pressure senses pleural pressure as its surrounding pressure, the change in diastolic pulmonary artery pressure will equal the change in pleural pressure. The ratio of the change in pleural pressure to change in airway pressure reflecting lung compliance can be considered an index of the transmission of the airway pressure to the pleural space. To calculate transmural Ppao, one merely subtracts the product of the index of transmission for PEEP (measured in mm Hg) from Ppao.[24] Because lung compliance varies little over the course of the day, one need only calculate the index of transmission once, so these estimates of transmural Ppao can be calculated each time Ppao is measured.

Although the general rule is that measurements should be made at end-expiration, this is not always the case. Normally expiration is passive so that pleural pressure does not deviate much from the baseline during expiration. However, dyspneic patients often expire actively, which raises pleural pressure, and this occurs with 2 patterns (**Fig. 5**). In one the patient pushes out from the start of expiration and, depending on the length of expiration, all the inspired air may or may not be expired during the period of expiration, which elevates pleural pressure and, consequently, intrathoracic vascular pressure relative to atmosphere. Furthermore, measured pressures will then vary with the length of expiration. The other pattern is more problematic. In this situation the patient pushes down progressively more during expiration so that there is a marked increase in pleural pressure at end-expiration. When this pattern is present, pressures should be measured at the beginning of expiration and before the patient starts pushing down. Major errors will occur in this situation if measurements are made at end-expiration. One also can try to identify a breath that occurs without active expiration. Asking a patient to talk (even if intubated) can be tried to temporarily stop active expiration, as active abdominal muscles usually do not contract when talking.

Another consideration is at which point in the cardiac cycle the pressure measurement should be taken on a right atrial tracing (**Figs. 6** and **7**). This issue becomes important when there are large "a" and "v" waves or prominent "x" or "y" descents. Because a primary use of atrial pressure is assessment of cardiac preload, the pressure measurement should be taken at the base of the "c" wave, called the "z" point, or if the "c" is not evident just after the QRS wave on the ECG. The rationale is that this is the final pressure at the end of diastole and before the onset of contraction, and thus is the best estimate of preload.

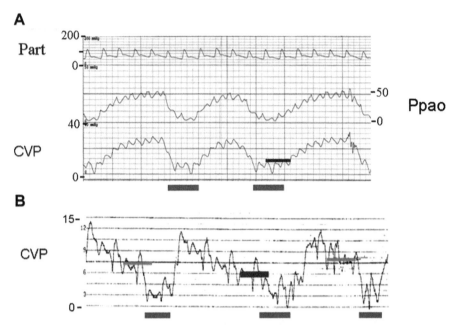

Fig. 5. (*A*) Example of a spontaneous effort with a marked active expiration with progressive increases in the pressures throughout expiration. The lines at the bottom indicate inspiration. The line on the CVP tracing suggests an appropriate place for the measurement; although it is early in expiration, it occurs before the major push. (*B*) Example of active expiration with a decrease in effort throughout the expiratory phase. The value at end-expiration in the middle breath is lower than the other 2 because the breath is longer and there is more time for expiration. (*Reproduced from* Magder S. Hemodynamic monitoring in the mechanically ventilated patient. Curr Opin Crit Care 2011;17(1):36–42.)

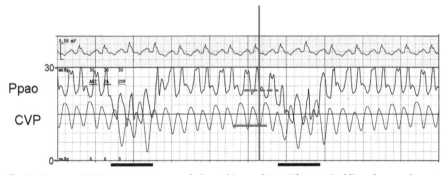

Fig. 6. Ppao and CVP in a spontaneously breathing subject. The vertical line shows where to make the measurement based on the QRS. The horizontal lines mark inspiration. The inspiratory decrease in Ppao is prominent, indicating a strong inspiratory effort, but there is only an increase in the "y" descent on the CVP with no change of the base of the "a" and "c" waves during inspiration (although there is a slight increase during expiration indicating some active expiration). Based on this pattern, it is unlikely that this patient would respond to fluid.

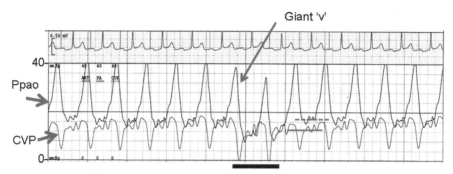

Fig. 7. Ppao and CVP in a spontaneously breathing subject. Giant "v" waves are evident on the Ppao tracing and there is a marked "y" descent. There is a slow rising "v" wave, suggesting limited left atrial compliance and prominent "y," indicating restriction on the right side. It is unlikely that this patient would respond to fluids. The thick bar marks inspiration, as is evident by the increase in the "y" descent on the CVP. There is slight forced expiration so that the Ppao (*dashed line*, 16 mm Hg) and CVP (*solid line*, 12 mm Hg) are not made at end-expiration.

Cardiac Output

Modern PAC injection setups have greatly reduced errors in the measurement of cardiac output by thermodilution. Helpful features include a syringe that only allows a fixed amount of volume, which is usually 10 mL of saline, valves that allow drawing the fluid from a bag and injecting without having to manually turn a valve, and a temperature probe that obtains the temperature of the injectate as it is goes into the patient. Precautions include ensuring that the exact amount of fluid is drawn up in the syringe, that the bolus is given quickly, and that the patient's baseline temperature in the blood is constant.[25] In this regard it is important to ensure that a large amount of another fluid is not being infused at the same time through another line, as this changes the baseline temperature and is the equivalent of adding extra indicator. After each injection the curves should be inspected on the monitor to ensure that there are no irregularities and that the downward curve is smooth (**Fig. 8**). It is not necessary to time injections to a phase of ventilation, because stroke volume does change during the ventilatory cycle and it is not possible to reach exactly the same point in the cycle. Repeated injections thus give an average value, which is also what the tissues see.

With the basic PAC, cardiac output is obtained by performing usually 3 or more injections of saline at room temperature, and taking the average of the 3 if the curves on the monitor look appropriate in that they have a clean rise and fall and are smooth. Devices are also available for continuous measurements of mixed venous oxygen saturation and continuous thermodilution cardiac output measures. The latter work by using transfer of heat from a filament mounted on the PAC close to the injection port at the level of the right ventricle, and the increase in temperature is sensed distally.[26] Repeated pseudorandom pulses of heat with different filament powers are used to reconstruct a thermodilution curve. The advantage of these devices is that trends are readily observed and provide earlier indications of significant changes. However, these continuous cardiac output devices are considerably more expensive than routine PAC, and their cost-effectiveness has not been demonstrated.[27] There are also some potential disadvantages. Variations in cardiac output and mixed venous oxygen saturation occur regularly because of biological variations such as changes in wakefulness, fever, or drug infusions, without there actually being a pathologic problem. There thus can be a tendency to overreact with these continuous cardiac output

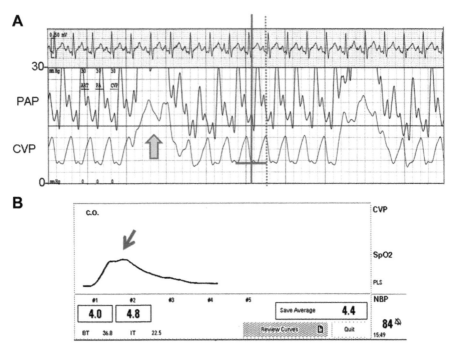

Fig. 8. (*A*) PAP and CVP tracings in a mechanically ventilated subject. The solid line shows how the electrocardiogram (ECG) can be used to time and identify the CVP waves. The prominent CVP wave (*arrow*) occurs after the QRS and is thus a prominent "v." The solid vertical line is drawn after the QRS and indicates a likely "c" wave, which is where CVP should be measured (*horizontal line*, 5 mm Hg). The vertical dotted line is drawn from the peak of "v" wave and appears late in the electrical cycle, indicating that in this case there is a significant delay between the electrical ECG signal and the fluid-based CVP and PAP signals. (*B*) Thermodilution cardiac output curve with a "notch" at the peak of the temperature curve (*arrow*) and variation in the measured cardiac outputs. There is a marked inspiratory increase in PAP and CVP in *A*, indicating that thoracic compliance is likely low. The consequent large increase in pleural pressure (>15 mm Hg) during inspiration interfered with the thermodilution curve. In support of this, the notch in the thermodilution curve was not present when the ventilator was paused (not shown).

devices. The averaging of values involved in the algorithm can sometimes fail to detect an increase in cardiac output following a fluid bolus because of the time needed for a change to be observed.[28]

Mixed Venous Oxygen Saturation

Mixed venous oxygen saturation is obtained by drawing blood from the distal end of the PAC and measuring the oxygen saturation with a co-oximeter, or in vivo by using a fiberoptic sensor at the tip of the PAC. When sampling mixed venous blood, it is important to ensure that the catheter is not wedged in the pulmonary artery or that blood is not withdrawn too quickly, as this will result in withdrawal of pulmonary capillary blood after gas exchange and thus render a falsely elevated O_2 saturation and decreased venous carbon dioxide pressure (PCO_2) value. Arterization of the mixed venous sample can be suspected when the mixed venous O_2 saturation is very high (ie, >80%). The PAC may be purposely wedged to obtain a "capillary" or left atrial equivalent sample if one wishes to calculate intrapulmonary shunt.

Approach to the Patient

Invasive hemodynamic monitoring comprises both arterial and central venous/PAC monitoring. Arterial catheterization is useful because it allows continuous monitoring of arterial pressure and its various components: systolic, diastolic, and pulse pressure, and pulse pressure variation during mechanical ventilation. The article by Pinsky on functional hemodynamic monitoring elsewhere in this issue focuses on arterial waveform analysis, so here the focus is on right-sided pressure and flow monitoring. One can approach the hemodynamic monitoring needs of the patient using data derived from the PAC, or with a less invasive measurement of cardiac output and CVP[8] using a central venous catheter.

The PAC is often used either as a diagnostic tool or for titration of therapy. A common diagnostic problem that can be assessed by data derived from the PAC is determination of the cause of hypotension. Blood pressure is approximately equal to the product of cardiac output and systemic arterial resistance. Resistance is a calculated variable based on the measurement of blood pressure and cardiac output. In the hypotensive patient, the initiating problem is the low blood pressure. Thus, measurement of cardiac output is key in the decision-making process. If cardiac output is normal or elevated then the primary reason for the low blood pressure is a decrease in systemic vascular resistance. The differential diagnosis is then clear, and the possibilities easily evaluated (**Box 1**). Of these, sepsis is by far the most likely commonly occurring cause seen in hospitalized patients. The most specific therapy for hypotension caused by low systemic vascular resistance is the use of a vasoconstrictor drug, such as norepinephrine, to increase vasomotor tone. However, using fluid boluses also can improve blood pressure if the heart is volume responsive by further increasing cardiac output, although this assumes that the volume-responsive heart is not functioning on the flat part of the cardiac function curve. Volume resuscitation increases cardiac output by

---

Box 1
Causes of decreases systemic vascular resistance

- Sepsis (systemic inflammatory response syndrome)
- Drugs (specifically drugs that actively dilate resistance vessels)
  - α-Antagonists
  - β-Agonists
  - Nitroprusside
  - Phosphodiesterase inhibitors (milrinone)
  - Hydralazine
- Spinal/epidural injections
- Spinal injury
- Cirrhosis
- Arterial-venous fistula
- Adrenal insufficiency
- Thyroid disease
- Anaphylaxis
- Anemia (severe, long-standing)
- Beriberi

increasing venous pressure, meaning that capillary pressures must also be increased, which will increase capillary leak, which is already increased in many of the causes of distributive shock.

When a hypotensive patient has a decreased cardiac output, low blood flow is the primary cause of hypotension. Because cardiac output is determined by the interaction of cardiac function and venous return, either of these can explain a decrease in cardiac output. Which of these two is the primary reason can be determined by examining CVP as a measure of right atrial pressure. In the presence of a low cardiac output, a low CVP argues for a primary venous return problem, whereas a high CVP argues for a primary cardiac problem. Trends in CVP and cardiac output are even more helpful. If the cardiac output decreased with a drop in CVP, the primary problem is a decrease in venous return, and cardiac output will most likely increase with a volume infusion. If the cardiac output decreased with an increase in CVP, the most likely problem is a decrease in pump function. Fluid is less likely to be of help, and attention should be turned to diagnosing the reason for the decrease in pump function and to increasing pump function. When it is not clear as to which is the culprit, a volume challenge can help distinguish between these two possibilities. A cardiac function problem may or may not respond to a volume infusion, but a venous return problem should always respond to a volume infusion. Thus, a failure of a volume bolus to increase cardiac output despite an increase in CVP indicates a cardiac limitation, and therapy should be directed at improving cardiac function.

There are two parts to monitoring patients. One is identifying the need to intervene because hemodynamic values are outside a desired range. These values can be set as goals for all patients in what is called goal-directed therapy, and implies a preventive approach, or according to set of triggers for specific interventions based on the patient's overall status, which implies a more responsive approach. Responsive approaches reflect traditional management principles, whereas goal-directed therapies represent which resuscitation targets that are empirically defined. Another article by Cannesson and colleagues elsewhere in this issue addresses goal-directed therapies and their logic. One form of goal-directed algorithms recommends giving fluids until the patient is no longer volume responsive. A recent clinical study supports the argument that this is not a good practice.[29] First, volume responsiveness does not indicate a volume need. Normal persons usually function on the ascending volume-responsive part of the cardiac function curve, thus allowing changes in both cardiac and return functions to regulate cardiac output. When the heart is functioning on the flat part of the cardiac function curve, only an increase in cardiac function can increase cardiac output, which is especially important when managing patients after heart transplantation. Because the transplanted heart is not innervated, changes in cardiac function require either secretion of adrenal catecholamines, which must arrive at the heart through the circulation, or intrinsic increases in contractility by the Anrep mechanism, both of which take minutes to realize. If the response is not sufficiently rapid to increase the cardiac output, the patient's condition can rapidly deteriorate.

The most common initial intervention in a hypotensive patient who is not bleeding or hypoxemic is the use of a fluid bolus. In an analysis of the use of fluid boluses in a recent study, the primary triggers were cardiac output or blood pressure below target.[30,31] The target value of CVP as a trigger for a volume bolus was set low and only rarely was a trigger, as was the case for urine output. In a responsive approach it is important to follow what happens after a fluid bolus is given. If the cardiac output or blood pressure triggers are corrected, nothing further needs to be done until they fall outside the desired range again. However, if they were not corrected, the next step is to determine whether the fluid challenge was adequate by determining if the CVP rose sufficiently to increase cardiac output by the Starling mechanism. An increase in CVP of 2 mm Hg or more is considered significant because this pressure change can be recognized on the monitor. If the CVP rises by at least 2 mm Hg and cardiac output increases but the blood pressure still is below the target, more fluid can be given. If the CVP rises by 2 mm Hg or more and cardiac output does not increase, this indicates that the heart is functioning on the flat part of the cardiac function curve and that further volume loading will not be helpful. It should be appreciated that if the plateau of the cardiac function curve occurs at a cardiac output of 5 L/min and a CVP of 10 mm Hg, the slope from a CVP of zero to 10 mm Hg is 0.5 L/min, which underestimates the steep part of the cardiac function curve. Thus an increase in CVP of 2 mm Hg should produce an observable increase in cardiac output if the heart is volume responsive. If the heart is not responsive to a volume infusion, correction of hypotension requires a vasopressor if the cardiac output is adequate or an inotrope if the cardiac output needs to be increased. Although norepinephrine is thought of as a vasopressor, it still produces some increase in cardiac contractility[32] and can serve both purposes if only smaller increases in cardiac output are needed.

Pulmonary Artery Occlusion Pressure

In the discussion so far on fluid management, Ppao has not been included because Ppao is useful for diagnostic purposes and the potential of pulmonary edema, but not for the determination of the need of fluid to increase cardiac output. CVP indicates the interaction of cardiac function and return function, and thus always is the appropriate value to use for separating these 2 functions. This point is especially important when there is right heart limitation, a common occurrence in both postoperative cardiac surgery and septic patients. When there is right heart limitation, changes in Ppao have little effect on cardiac output, as the left heart only can put out what the right heart gives it. However, the value of Ppao allows distinction of a primary left heart versus right heart cause of a decrease in cardiac function. This rationale was the original one of Swan and Ganz when they developed the PAC.[33,34] Swan worked in a coronary care unit where left ventricular dysfunction without right ventricular dysfunction is common and not easily recognized with just CVP and cardiac output measurements. The failing left ventricle tends to produce more pulmonary edema with moderate decreases in cardiac output and little change in CVP. If Ppao is much more elevated than the CVP, the differential diagnosis favors left heart failure as the primary disease process. The problem must be due to a marked increase in left ventricular load (hypertension), aortic or mitral valve disease, or ischemic heart disease. And if Ppao rises high enough, there should also be pulmonary edema. By contrast, a generalized cardiomyopathy should affect both ventricles, and the failing right ventricle protects the left ventricle. The pertinent phrase is: no left ventricular failure without right ventricular success.

Ppao also gives an indication of the potential for pulmonary edema, especially when there is a capillary leak syndrome, although it has been shown not to be as good as an actual measurement of lung water.[35,36] An important potential artifact that can occur in measuring Ppao is failure to actually obtain an occlusion of the vessel but instead only dampening the pulmonary artery pressure (see **Fig. 4**). This artifact should be considered when the Ppao is the same as the pulmonary artery diastolic pressure, especially when there is an elevated pulmonary artery pressure. The wave pattern of the Ppao also can be helpful. Large "v" waves are suggestive of mitral regurgitation (see **Fig. 7**; **Fig. 9**). In severe, acute mitral regurgitation this even can look like a pulmonary artery tracing. However, large "v" waves also can be produced by overfilling of the left

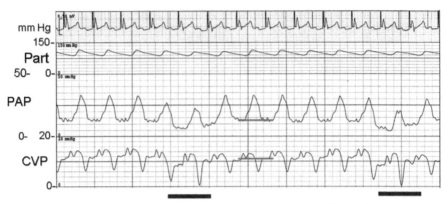

Fig. 9. Arterial (Part), distal pulmonary artery catheter pressure (PAP), and CVP in spontaneously breathing subject. The PAP tracing is actually a large "v" wave from a Ppao occlusion. Note the slow upstroke of the wave compared with the PAP examples in **Figs. 3** and **4**. There was + to ++ mitral regurgitation on echocardiography. The "v" wave increased overnight after volume loading. The "y" descent is prominent, indicating likely RV limitation. The horizontal lines indicate inspiration. There is a mild active expiration (increase in CVP during expiration). The rhythm (*upper band*) is atrial paced.

heart because of excess volume. This pattern often is seen in patients who have a ventricular septal defect or rupture in association with an acute myocardial infection.

Pulmonary Artery Pressure

Pulmonary artery pressure gives an indication of the load on the right heart. Based on the approach of Wood,[37] mechanisms of pulmonary hypertension can be classified as the following: (1) passive pulmonary hypertension whereby the rise in pressure is due to increased left-sided diastolic pressure; (2) reactive pulmonary hypertension, which is due to changes in pulmonary vascular resistance because of persistent high pulmonary blood flow, as occurs with left to right cardiac shunts or chronic hypoxia; (3) obliterative pulmonary hypertension attributable to loss of the pulmonary vascular cross-sectional area that can be due to pulmonary embolic disease or vascular destruction from inflammatory or fibrotic processes; (4) primary pulmonary vascular disease caused by disease processes that directly target the pulmonary vasculature, including primary pulmonary hypertension. An elevated pulmonary artery pressure itself does not indicate the stress on the right heart, as the pressure is related to the cardiac output and the resistance. How well the right heart is coping with the elevated pressure can be evaluated by observing the cardiac output and CVP. If the CVP is low and cardiac output is normal, the right heart is tolerating the increased load. An increase in CVP and a decrease in cardiac output is a bad prognostic sign.

Mixed Venous Oxygen and Consumption of Oxygen

Presence of a PAC also allows sampling of mixed venous O_2 saturation from the pulmonary artery. Although directly targeting therapy based on mixed venous blood values has not been shown to be helpful and possibly harmful,[38] the addition of this measurement can be used to support other measurements. For example, a decrease in cardiac output would be expected to be associated with a decrease in mixed venous O_2 and an increase in lactate in patients who are in circulatory shock, and these then can be used to support the validity of an observed decrease.[38] Alternatively, if the patient has a low cardiac output but the mixed venous O_2 saturation is

70% and the lactate concentration is normal, the cardiac output likely is sufficient for the patient's needs, and observation rather than intervention might be the best approach. Although one should not treat an isolated low mixed venous O_2 saturation value, it should also not be dismissed. Interpretation needs to be based on the whole picture, including the actual cardiac output value, organ function, and metabolic status as indicated by lactate.

A useful way of confirming that the measured values make sense is to calculate the oxygen consumption by using the indirect Fick method from the cardiac output, Hgb, and the arterial and venous saturations (use fractions instead of percentages to make the units work).

$$Vo_2 = \text{Cardiac output (L/min)} \times \text{Hgb (g/L)} \times 1.36 \times \text{(arterial-venous } O_2 \text{ saturation)}$$

The value is in mL/min and 1.36 is the amount of O_2 per gram of hemoglobin. Typical values are in the 200 to 300 mL/min range depending on body size and resting metabolic activity. If the calculated value is too high or too low for the patient, the components should be examined to determine which values likely are incorrect.

Nonhemodynamic Uses of Invasive Pressure Measurements

Because the heart is surrounded by pleural pressure, intracardiac pressures change with changes in pleural pressure. Both right and left atrial pressures increase and decrease with pleural pressure, but the relationship of change in left atrial pressure (referenced relative to atmosphere) to change in pleural pressure is much closer than in the right atrium, because when the venous return curve intersects the ascending part of the cardiac function curve, a decrease in pleural pressure lowers right atrial pressure relative to atmosphere and increases right heart filling. However, when the right heart is on the flat part of the cardiac function curve, the right atrial pressure does not decrease with a spontaneous inspiration because cardiac filling cannot be increased by the drop in pleural pressure (see **Figs. 6** and **9; Fig. 10**). Even a trivial increase in right ventricular volume immediately brings the CVP back to baseline. This process can be used to indicate whether the heart will or will not respond to volume.[39] The drop in pleural pressure can be recognized by an increase in the magnitude of the "y" descent, which then can be used to "mark" the inspiratory effort (see **Figs. 6, 7, 9,** and **10**).

In contrast to what happens with the right heart, the reservoir filling the left heart, the pulmonary venous compartment, also is in the chest, so that its pressure and that of the left atrium decrease together and the pressure gradient filling the left heart does not change with the drop in pleural pressure. Respiratory changes in Ppao thus track

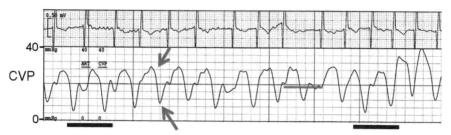

Fig. 10. CVP in subject with a restrictive cardiomyopathy (myocardial fibroelastosis) breathing spontaneously. The "v" wave (*downward arrow*) is broad, indicating tricuspid regurgitation, and so is the deep "y" descent (*upward arrow*), owing to the restrictive cardiomyopathy. The horizontal lines mark inspiration. The rhythm is atrial fibrillation.

changes in pleural pressure very well[40] and can be used to assess inspiratory changes in pleural pressure. The decrease in Ppao with inspiration is slightly less than the decrease in pleural pressure as measured by an esophageal balloon, because lung inflation usually slightly increases left heart filling by squeezing blood out of the alveolar vessels. This process slightly increases left atrial transmural pressure during inspiration.[41]

Inspiratory swings in CVP and Ppao during positive pressure ventilation also can give an indication that thoracic compliance is decreased, which includes the chest and abdomen. When thoracic compliance is decreased, the increase in pleural pressure for the same tidal volume is larger; this is evidenced by larger than normal increases in CVP and Ppao during inspirations with normal tidal volumes (see **Fig. 8**).

The magnitude of the "y" descent on the CVP, an indication of early ventricular filling, also can be helpful. A large "y" descent (ie, >4 mm Hg) is suggestive of restrictive conditions (see **Figs. 7, 9**, and **10**), meaning that the heart is functioning on the flat part of the cardiac function curve and that it is unlikely that a volume infusion will increase cardiac output.[12] Loss of "y" descents is seen when there is cardiac tamponade and, in the face of a decrease in cardiac output and blood pressure, indicates the need for an intervention to decompress the heart.

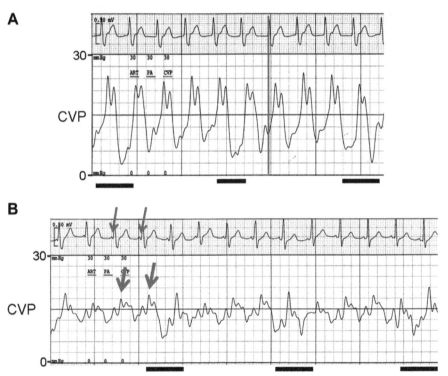

Fig. 11. CVP tracing from subject with junctional rhythm. The rhythm is regular and there are no "p" waves. (*A*) The prominent waves in the CVP tracing are cannon "a" waves caused by retrograde "p" waves and atrial contractions during systole. In (*B*) atrial activity is evident (*arrows*) but the PR interval is short, indicating a low atrial or junctional focus. The "a" waves are much smaller and increase at the end of inspiration. The subject had emergency mitral valve replacement after inferior wall myocardial infarction and ruptured papillary muscle.

Another potential use of pressure waveforms is to interpret rhythms on the ECG. An example of retrograde "p" waves producing cannon "a" wave on the CVP tracing is shown in **Fig. 11.**

SUMMARY

Almost 20 years ago an observational study by Connors and colleagues[42] started a debate on the use of the PAC, which many thought would lead to its extinction. However, the PAC is still in use and in selected situations can give much useful information at a lower cost than other devices. Proper use of a PAC requires an understanding of principles of measurements, attention to safety concerns, and, above all, a good understanding of the regulation of cardiac output. If one exerts the effort to master its use, it can be a valuable tool for the management of complex hemodynamic problems.

REFERENCES

1. Rajaram SS, Desai NK, Kalra A, et al. Pulmonary artery catheters for adult patients in intensive care. Cochrane Database Syst Rev 2013;(2):CD003408.
2. Richard C, Warszawski J, Anguel N, et al. Early use of the pulmonary artery catheter and outcomes in patients with shock and acute respiratory distress syndrome: a randomized controlled trial. JAMA 2003;290(20):2713–20.
3. Harvey S, Harrison DA, Singer M, et al. Assessment of the clinical effectiveness of pulmonary artery catheters in management of patients in intensive care (PAC-Man): a randomised controlled trial. Lancet 2005;366(9484):472–7.
4. Sandham JD, Hull RD, Brant RF, et al. A randomized, controlled trial of the use of pulmonary-artery catheters in high-risk surgical patients. N Engl J Med 2003; 348(1):5–14.
5. Wheeler AP, Bernard GR, Thompson BT, et al. Pulmonary-artery versus central venous catheter to guide treatment of acute lung injury. N Engl J Med 2006; 354(21):2213–24.
6. Iberti TJ, Fisher EP, Leibowitz AB, et al. A multicenter study of physicians' knowledge of the pulmonary artery catheter. Pulmonary artery catheter study group. JAMA 1990;264(22):2928–32.
7. Iberti TJ, Daily EK, Leibowitz AB, et al. Assessment of critical care nurses' knowledge of the pulmonary artery catheter. The pulmonary artery catheter study group. Crit Care Med 1994;10:1674–8.
8. Magder S. An approach to hemodynamic monitoring: Guyton at the beside. Crit Care 2012;16:236–43.
9. Magder S, Scharf SM. Venous return. In: Scharf SM, Pinsky MR, Magder SA, editors. Respiratory-circulatory interactions in health and disease. 2nd edition. New York: Marcel Dekker, Inc; 2001. p. 93–112.
10. Rothe C. Venous system: physiology of the capacitance vessels. In: Shepherd JT, Abboud FM, editors. Handbook of physiology. Bethesda (MD): American Physiologic Society; 1983. p. 397–452.
11. Bishop VS, Stone HL, Guyton AC. Cardiac function curves in conscious dogs. Am J Physiol 1964;207(3):677–82.
12. Magder S, Bafaqeeh F. The clinical role of central venous pressure measurements. J Intensive Care Med 2007;22(1):44–51.
13. Magder S, De Varennes B. Clinical death and the measurement of stressed vascular volume. Crit Care Med 1998;26:1061–4.

14. Deschamps A, Magder S. Baroreflex control of regional capacitance and blood flow distribution with or without alpha adrenergic blockade. Am J Physiol 1992; 263:H1755–63.
15. Magder S. Theoretical analysis of the non-cardiac limits to maximum exercise. Can J Physiol Pharmacol 2002;80:971–9.
16. Magder S. Heart-lung interactions in sepsis. In: Scharf SM, Pinsky M, Magder S, editors. Respiratory-circulatory interactions in health and disease. 2nd edition. New York: Marcel Dekker, Inc; 2001. p. 739–62.
17. O'Grady NP, Alexander M, Burns LA, et al. Guidelines for the prevention of intravascular catheter-related infections. Am J Infect Control 2011;39(4 Suppl 1):S1–34.
18. Mermel LA, Maki DG. Infectious complications of Swan-Ganz pulmonary artery catheters. Pathogenesis, epidemiology, prevention, and management. Am J Respir Crit Care Med 1994;149(4 Pt 1):1020–36.
19. Magder S. Hemodynamic monitoring in the mechanically ventilated patient. Curr Opin Crit Care 2011;17(1):36–42.
20. Magder SA. The highs and lows of blood pressure: toward meaningful clinical targets in patients with shock. Crit Care Med 2014;42(5):1241–51.
21. Magder S. Central venous pressure: a useful but not so simple measurement. Crit Care Med 2006;34(8):2224–7.
22. Magder S. Mechanical interactions between the respiratory and circulatory systems. In: Bradley TD, Floras JS, editors. Sleep apnea: implications in cardiovascular and cerebrovascular disease. 2nd edition. New York: Informa Health Care USA, Inc; 2010. p. 40–60.
23. Carter RS, Snyder JV, Pinsky MR. LV filling pressure during PEEP measured by nadir wedge pressure after airway disconnection. Am J Physiol 1985;249(4 Pt 2):H770–6.
24. Teboul JL, Pinsky MR, Mercat A, et al. Estimating cardiac filling pressure in mechanically ventilated patients with hyperinflation. Crit Care Med 2000;28(11): 3631–6.
25. Magder S. Cardiac output measurement. In: Tobin MJ, editor. Principles and practice of intensive care monitoring. Chicago: McGraw-Hill; 1997. p. 797–810.
26. Cariou A, Monchi M, Dhainaut JF. Continuous cardiac output and mixed venous oxygen saturation monitoring. J Crit Care 1998;13(4):198–213.
27. Medin DL, Brown DT, Wesley R, et al. Validation of continuous thermodilution cardiac output in critically ill patients with analysis of systematic errors. J Crit Care 1998;13(4):184–9.
28. Critchley LA, Lee A, Ho AM. A critical review of the ability of continuous cardiac output monitors to measure trends in cardiac output. Anesth Analg 2010;111(5): 1180–92.
29. Challand C, Struthers R, Sneyd JR, et al. Randomized controlled trial of intraoperative goal-directed fluid therapy in aerobically fit and unfit patients having major colorectal surgery. Br J Anaesth 2012;108(1):53–62.
30. Magder S, Potter BJ, Varennes BD, et al. Fluids after cardiac surgery: a pilot study of the use of colloids versus crystalloids. Crit Care Med 2010;38(11): 2117–24.
31. Potter BJ, Deverenne B, Doucette S, et al. Cardiac output responses in a flow-driven protocol of resuscitation following cardiac surgery. J Crit Care 2013; 28(3):265–9.
32. Datta P, Magder S. Hemodynamic response to norepinephrine with and without inhibition of nitric oxide synthase in porcine endotoxemia. Am J Respir Crit Care Med 1999;160(6):1987–93.

33. Swan HJ, Ganz W, Forrester J, et al. Catheterization of the heart in man with use of a flow-directed balloon-tipped catheter. N Engl J Med 1970;282(9):447–51.
34. Forrester JS, Diamond G, McHugh TJ, et al. Filling pressures in the right and left sides of the heart in acute myocardial infarction. A reappraisal of central-venous-pressure monitoring. N Engl J Med 1971;285(4):190–3.
35. Schuller D, Schuster DP. Fluid-management strategies in acute lung injury. N Engl J Med 2006;355(11):1175.
36. Mitchell JP, Schuller D, Calandrino FS, et al. Improved outcome based on fluid management in critically ill patients requiring pulmonary artery catheterization. Am Rev Respir Dis 1992;145(5):990–8.
37. Wood P. Pulmonary hypertension. Br Med Bull 1952;8(4):348–53.
38. Gattinoni L, Brazzi L, Pelosi P, et al. A trial of goal-oriented hemodynamic therapy in critically ill patients. SvO_2 Collaborative Group. N Engl J Med 1995;333(16): 1025–32.
39. Magder S, Lagonidis D, Erice F. The use of respiratory variations in right atrial pressure to predict the cardiac output response to PEEP. J Crit Care 2002; 16(3):108–14.
40. Bellemare P, Goldberg P, Magder S. Variations in pulmonary artery occlusion pressure to estimate changes in pleural pressure. Intensive Care Med 2007; 33(11):2004–8.
41. Magder SA, Lichtenstein S, Adelman AG. Effects of negative pleural pressure on left ventricular hemodynamics. Am J Cardiol 1983;52(5):588–93.
42. Connors AF Jr, Speroff T, Dawson NV. The effectiveness of right heart catheterization in the initial care of critically ill patients. JAMA 1996;18:1294–5.

Functional Hemodynamic Monitoring

Michael R. Pinsky, MD, CM, Dr hc, MCCM

KEYWORDS

- Functional hemodynamic monitoring • Dynamic tissue O_2 saturation
- Positive-pressure ventilation • Stroke volume variation

KEY POINTS

- Functional hemodynamic monitoring reflects the assessment of the dynamic interactions of hemodynamic variables in response to a defined perturbation.
- Dynamic tissue O_2 saturation responses to complete stop-flow conditions (vascular occlusion test) assess cardiovascular sufficiency and distribution of microcirculatory blood flow.
- Dynamic inspiratory changes in central venous pressure during spontaneous ventilation identify both cor pulmonale and volume responsiveness.
- Dynamic changes in arterial pulse pressure (diastole to systole) and left ventricular stroke volume during positive-pressure ventilation reflect the degree to which the subject is volume responsive.
- Both pulse pressure variation (PPV) and stroke volume variation (SVV) quantitatively track volume responsiveness, with a threshold value of greater than 10% to 15% defining a subject whose cardiac output will increase by greater than 15% in response to a 500-mL fluid bolus.
- Dynamic changes in PPV and SVV cannot be used in the setting of atrial fibrillation, acute cor pulmonale, or when spontaneous breathing is forceful and erratic.
- Dynamic changes in cardiac output in response to a passive leg-raising maneuver also predict volume responsiveness.
- PPV/SVV defines central arterial stiffness or elastance, and can be used as a surrogate marker of vasomotor tone.

This work was supported in part by the National Institutes of Health grants HL67181 and HL073198.

Potential Conflicts of Interest: M.R. Pinsky is the inventor of a University of Pittsburgh US Patent "Use of aortic pulse pressure and flow in bedside hemodynamic management." Member of the Scientific Advisory Board for LiDCO Ltd. Stock options from LiDCO Ltd and Cheetah Medical, Ltd.

Receives institutional funding for research from Edwards LifeSciences, Inc.

Department of Critical Care Medicine, University of Pittsburgh, 606 Scaife Hall, 3550 Terrace Street, Pittsburgh, PA 15261, USA

E-mail address: pinskymr@upmc.edu

Crit Care Clin 31 (2015) 89–111

http://dx.doi.org/10.1016/j.ccc.2014.08.005

criticalcare.theclinics.com

0749-0704/15/$ – see front matter © 2015 Elsevier Inc. All rights reserved.

INTRODUCTION

Hemodynamic monitoring is the active assessment of cardiopulmonary status by the use of biosensors that assess physiologic outputs. The simplest form of monitoring is the individual health care professional, inspecting the patient for consciousness, agitation or distress, breathing regular or labored, the presence or absence of central and peripheral cyanosis; touching of the skin of a patient to note if it is cool and moist, and if capillary refill is rapid or not; palpation of the central and peripheral pulses to note rate and firmness.

Although well established and important as bedside diagnostic tools, these simple "human-instrument" measures can be greatly expanded by the use of pulse oximetry to estimate arterial oxygen saturation (Spo_2), and the sphygmomanometer and auscultation to note systolic and diastolic blood pressure and identify pulsus paradoxus. These classic measures of hemodynamics, often referred to as routine vital signs, are central to the assessment of cardiorespiratory sufficiency and much of diagnostic bedside medicine is rooted in these important techniques.

However, with some exceptions, these simple and inexpensive measures do not have the discriminatory value in identifying patients as being stable or unstable when compensatory processes mask instability or when changes in physiologic state occur rapidly. Furthermore, they predict poorly who are at an early stage of an instability process, such as hypovolemia or heart failure, but compensating. Within the context of circulatory shock, tachycardia may or may not develop early and even if it is present, it is nonspecific. However, these simple measures can be markedly helped in their sensitivity to detect effective hypovolemia by making these same measures before and during an orthostatic challenge. For example, measuring blood pressure and pulse rate changes between lying supine, sitting, and standing markedly increase the diagnostic capability of the measures to identify functional hypovolemia. If heart rate increases and/or blood pressure decreases with sitting or standing, it is reasonable to presume that some degree of compatible hypovolemia exists. However, the other important concept in making these observations is that the measures themselves do not change, but their measured values change in response to a defined physiologic challenge: this is an example of functional hemodynamic monitoring.[1] Functional hemodynamic monitoring is the use of a defined physiologic stressor to access the physiologic reserve of the system.

Another example of functional hemodynamic monitoring is to use the morphology of the normal lead II electrocardiogram (ECG) to define ischemic heart disease. In practice, unless there is ongoing ischemia or prior infarction, the rhythm and morphology of the ECG signal is a poor marker of clinically relevant coronary artery disease. However, that same ECG signal, if monitoring during an exercise challenge that increases heart rate above a minimal amount defined by subject age, does not show any morphologic changes or arrhythmias, then it is highly unlikely that the subject has clinically significant coronary artery disease. It is important that as with the measure of pulse rate and blood pressure, ECG monitoring has not changed; it is the intervention that creates evolving hemodynamic parameters that markedly increase the sensitivity and specificity of hemodynamic monitoring to define cardiovascular state.

Using the functional hemodynamic monitoring principles described herein, it is possible for the bedside clinician to answer 4 interrelated and important questions of their patient[2]:

- Are they in compensated shock?
- Are they volume responsive?

- Is their arterial tone increased, normal, or decreased?
- Is their heart able to sustain flow without high filling pressures?

Although the examples herein reflect well-validated approaches to address each of these clinically relevant questions, they are neither complete nor exhaustive in their number and applications. Indeed, identifying novel functional parameters to define physiologic state, be it neurologic reserve, respiratory function, renal filtering, or gut absorption, reflect evolving frontiers of this approach across critical care disciplines. New indices of bodily functional reserve are constantly being identified, and the actual number of such potential indices is vast. The major issue going forward will not be the sensitivity or specificity of any new index, because most are fairly sensitive and specific, but the ease to which they can be assessed continuously or repeatedly in addition to their level of invasiveness. However, the examples given in this article have been proved to be robust and easily used parameters of physiologic reserve, and can be used as templates in validating and applying novel future indices.

EARLY IDENTIFICATION OF COMPENSATED SHOCK

It is difficult to identify patients early on in the course of circulatory shock because normal sympathetically medicated compensatory reflex mechanisms express themselves so as to sustain a relatively normal organ perfusion pressure and blood flow. For example, the normal response of the body to hypovolemia or impaired ventricular pump function is to attempt to maintain an adequate mean arterial pressure (MAP) by increasing sympathetic tone causing vasoconstriction, decreasing unstressed vascular volume, increased contractility, and tachycardia. In a healthy athlete early on in hypovolemic shock, tachycardia may not present, and in the elderly and those with dysautonomia tachycardia may not develop at all. Because these reflex sympathetic feedback mechanisms aim to sustain MAP above a minimal value to maintain cerebral and coronary blood flow, and because vascular capacitance is reduced to sustain cardiac output, hypotension not only occurs late but must be associated with tissue hypoperfusion. Hypotension in the setting of circulatory shock must also reflect failure of intrinsic compensatory mechanisms to sustain normal homeostasis. Thus, hypotension is a medical emergency not only because it must be associated with tissue hypoperfusion but also because it signals loss of intrinsic mechanisms to sustain effective blood flow. Furthermore, restoring MAP by the use of vasopressors improves tissue oxygenation in septic patients.[3] Thus, the immediate restoration of MAP while other flow-directed resuscitation efforts are under way is essential in minimizing ongoing tissue hypoperfusion.

Thus, if the bedside clinician waits for the patient to develop hypotension before treating cardiovascular insufficiency, some level of organ hypoperfusion must also coexist. Most goal-directed therapy resuscitation protocols show that prevention of tissue hypoperfusion by targeted hyper resuscitation before developing hypovolemia is associated with improved outcomes.[4] Biosensors and maneuvers that identify occult circulatory shock will be of importance in identifying those subjects at risk for hypoperfusion before severe tissue hypoperfusion develops. Furthermore, if their alarms trigger focused resuscitation efforts to prevent tissue hypoperfusion, improved outcome may also be realized as long as the primary cause of the hypoperfusion is also addressed. For example, early identification of occult hypovolemia associated with gastrointestinal hemorrhage will allow earlier fluid resuscitation but may not improve outcome if the cause of the hemorrhage is not also addressed. However, because cardiovascular insufficiency is characterized by an inadequate O_2 delivery relative to the metabolic demands, some level of decreased cardiovascular reserve must also be present in the early stages of shock. Because progressive hypovolemia can be initially compensated by autonomic mechanisms, regional vasoconstriction should be a common characteristic of compensated or early shock before the development of hypotension. In this stage of compensated shock, microcirculatory O_2 use, like arterial pressure or cardiac output, is often normal as the compensatory mechanism effectively sustains tissue O_2 delivery above a crisis level. However, microcirculation alterations in muscle and skin blood flow already occur in these early stages of shock because these vascular beds have high concentrations of α-adrenergic receptors. Moreover, resuscitation restores microcirculatory flow in a directionally similar fashion to the increases in cardiac output.[5] Thus, measures of tissue cardiovascular reserve should be a sensitive early warning measure of impending cardiovascular collapse. One method to assess the microcirculatory status is the noninvasive measurement of tissue oxygen saturation (Sto_2).

Noninvasive Measures of Oxygen Delivery Sufficiency

A fundamental unanswered question in shock resuscitation is the level of tissue perfusion and tissue wellness. Resuscitation of shock patients is one of the most challenging aspects of acute care medicine in regard to determining an optimal resuscitation end point, as patients may have inadequate regional tissue O_2 delivery despite apparent adequate systemic perfusion. Traditional end points of resuscitation, including targeting a minimal MAP, normalization of arterial base deficit or lactate, increased urine output, or restoration of mixed venous O_2 saturation (Svo_2) or central venous O_2 saturation ($Scvo_2$) to some minimal value carry inherent flaws in their application and practicality. In addition, many patients who are thought to be fully resuscitated, as defined by achieving a target MAP, have markedly reduced intravascular volume, a condition known as underresuscitated shock. If not resuscitated further, these patients develop progressive ischemic tissue injury and, eventually, organ failure and death. This state is commonly seen in trauma victims who initially respond to small-volume fluid resuscitation, but if not further resuscitated have an extremely high incidence of end-organ injury and death. If noninvasive measures of tissue O_2 delivery sufficiency could be made, these underresuscitated patents could be readily identified and treated.

Noninvasive measurement of Sto_2 using near-infrared spectroscopy (NIRS) is an accurate and valid method for the assessment of regional tissue O_2 saturation under local sampling volume of the sensing probe. NIRS has been used to assess the adequacy of cerebral, renal, and muscle blood flow by measuring local Sto_2. Regrettably, absolute Sto_2 values are of limited discriminating capacity because Sto_2 remains within the normal range until tissue hypoperfusion is fairly advanced. However, the addition of a dynamic ischemic challenge and noting the local response to that challenge has proved useful in exposing early cardiovascular stress. Although Sto_2 values do not decrease until tissue perfusion is very low, this measure becomes more sensitive and specific when monitoring the change in Sto_2 in response to a vascular occlusion test (VOT).

The VOT is a functional hemodynamic monitoring approach to uncovering problems in baseline blood flow distribution and cardiovascular reserve. The VOT Sto_2 waveform is shown in **Fig. 1**. If the Sto_2 probe is placed on the thenar eminence and a downstream arm blood pressure cuff is inflated to a pressure in excess of systolic arterial pressure, one can assess the effects of total vascular occlusion–induced tissue ischemia and release on downstream Sto_2. Sto_2 is measured on the thenar eminence, and transient rapid vascular occlusion of the arm by sphygmomanometer inflation to 20 mm Hg above systolic pressure is performed either for a defined time interval,

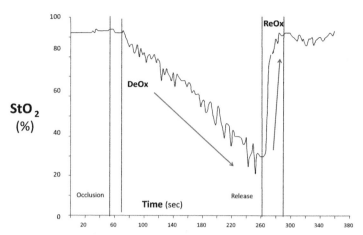

Fig. 1. Stylized display of the raw tissue oxygen saturation (Sto_2) trend during a vascular occlusion test. The initial vertical line connotes the start of vascular occlusion, whereas the second vertical line identifies when Sto_2 starts to decrease. The rate of decrease in Sto_2 or deoxygenation rate (DeOx) is defined by the mean slope of the initial decrease in Sto_2 following vascular occlusion (*blue arrow*). The third vertical line defines the point when the vascular occluder is released and forearm blood flow is resumes. The washout of deoxygenated blood causing reoxygenation (ReOx) is the second slope of the test (*red arrow*). (*Modified from* Gómez H, Torres A, Polanco P, et al. Use of noninvasive NIRS during a vascular occlusion test to assess dynamic tissue O(2) saturation response. Intensive Care Med 2008;34:1600–7.)

usually 3 minutes, or until Sto_2 declines to some threshold minimal value, usually 40%. This minimal Sto_2 value is presumed to induce a maximal level of local vasodilation, after which the vascular cuff is rapidly deflated to allow vascular reflow and washout of the deoxygenated blood from the downstream vascular beds. Several important parameters emerge from the VOT. The Sto_2 downslope, or deoxygenation rate (Dxo_2), reflects the local metabolic rate and effective local blood flow distribution. The Sto_2 recovery, or reoxygenation rate (Rxo_2), reflects local cardiovascular reserve and microcirculatory flow, as validated in trauma and septic patients in comparison with normal volunteers.[6]

Deoxygenation
The DeOx slope will increase if local metabolic rate increases, as will occur with contraction of the thenar muscles.[6] The DeOx slope will decrease if local metabolic rate decreases, but as it is difficult to decrease resting skeletal muscle oxygen consumption unless hypothermia exists; decreases in the DeOx slope usually reflect prior loss of vascular autoregulatory control. If before inducing total vascular occlusion the thenar vascular displayed a vasoplegic state, blood flow would become more uniform, thus increasing blood flow to capillary networks with a low intrinsic metabolic rate to levels similar to those beds with higher metabolic rates. The flow to the tissues with a higher metabolic rate would still be adequate, but "wasted" perfusion would result in a higher end-capillary pressure of O_2 than would otherwise be the case if flow were only proportional to metabolic need. On a macroscopic level, this is the presumed reason for the high mixed venous O_2 saturation (Svo_2) in hyperdynamic hypotensive septic shock. Thus, following regional vascular occlusion the regional Sto_2 of normally perfused capillary beds would decrease at its normal deoxygenation rate, whereas those with excessive flow for their metabolic needs would decrease more slowly.

The Sto_2 probe measures a mean Sto_2 for the entire bed, thus it would report a DeOx slower than would otherwise be the case. Thus, the slower the DeOx rate, presumably the greater the degree of vascular paralysis.

Reoxygenation

The ReOx reflects local vascular reserve. Because the occlusion causes global Sto_2 to decrease to a very low value (ie, 40%), local hypoxic vasodilation becomes maximal such that the ReOx rate will reflect only inflow rate of oxygenation blood. If vascular tone upstream from the site of vascular occlusion (usually the forearm) is increased, then despite removing the downstream occlusion the inflow of oxygenated blood will be less rapid, decreasing the rate of washout or ReOx. Indeed, both a decrease in DeOx in sepsis and a decrease in ReOx before fluid resuscitation have been reported in patients with septic shock.

The hypothesis that the alterations in VOT Sto_2 response are related to the outcome has been proved in patients with either severe sepsis or septic shock by Creteur and colleagues.[7] Furthermore, when compared with hemodynamically stable patients without infection (controls) and healthy volunteers, the differences in septic patients were striking. Using the Sto_2 VOT, Creteur and colleagues[7] assessed ReOx in addition to the difference between the maximum Sto_2 and the Sto_2 baseline as a measure of reactive hyperemia. Both the slope of ReOx and the overshoot were significantly lower in septic patients than in controls and healthy volunteers. The DeOx slopes were also significantly lower in the septic shock patients with cardiovascular insufficiency. ReOx slopes were higher in survivors than in nonsurvivors, and also tended to increase during resuscitation only in survivors. Finally, the ReOx slope was found to be a good predictor of ICU death. These differences between survivors and nonsurvivors were independent of MAP or vasopressor therapy.[7] These data suggest that the alterations in VOT Sto_2 ReOx are related more to the sepsis process itself and its severity than to organ perfusion pressure (MAP) or vasomotor tone (vasopressor therapy). If ReOx slope reflects inadequate local cardiovascular reserve, it should also be sensitive for an impending cardiovascular insufficiency state (compensated shock) if matched with other static measures of tissue ischemia.

Microcirculatory failure during shock is also thought to be a major component of the associated end-organ dysfunction.[8] Such microcirculatory dysfunction can be characterized by oxygen shunting, vasoconstriction, thrombosis, and tissue edema. As a result of these combined microcirculatory events, the flow distribution within the tissue is impaired. These microcirculatory alterations improve rapidly in survivors of septic shock, whereas patients dying by organ failure have a lower percentage of perfused small vessels.[9]

Predicting Outcome from Septic Shock

Mesquida and colleagues[10] took this approach one step further and explored whether Sto_2 VOT was a predictor of tissue hypoperfusion and organ injury using the Sequential Organ Failure Assessment (SOFA) score as a maker of organ injury. These investigators studied 33 patients with septic shock following restoration of MAP. Baseline Sto_2 was 76% ± 1% and were not different from values reported for normal controls. MAP correlated with both DeOx and ReOx slopes, consistent with known better tissue perfusion associated with high MAP in septic patients. However, after 24 hours only 17 patients had improved SOFA scores, consistent with improved organ system function, whereas the 18 other patients who did not demonstrate improved SOFA scores showed a persistently flattened DeOx slope consistent with persistent vasoplegia, and both DeOx and ReOx slopes impairments correlated with longer stays in the intensive care unit (ICU). Thus, by using a simple VOT, the NIRS StO_2 measure creates DeOx and ReOx parameters defining effective tissue blood flow.

Predicting the Need for Life-Saving Interventions

Perhaps more convincingly, Guyette and colleagues[11] showed that the StO_2 DeOx was able to predict the subsequent need for life-saving interventions (LSI) in STAT MedEvac air transport of trauma patients being transported to a Level 1 trauma center. These investigators assessed the predictive value of lactate and the StO_2 VOT in trauma patients during emergency air transport to the hospital from an accident site, usually a motor vehicle accident. All patients were monitored using 3-lead ECG, noninvasive blood pressure, heart rate, pulse oximeter O_2 saturation (SpO_2), and, when intubated, end-tidal CO_2 capnography. Previous work has documented that these single vital signs are not sensitive at identifying shock until they are advanced.[12] Because protocol-based algorithms typically rely on individual vital signs or clinical parameters (ie, cyanosis, altered mental status) to identify the need for LSI,[13,14] robust parameters of impending instability are important for the acute care triage of this salvageable critically ill trauma population. Subjective measures such as acute changes in mental status may be used to identify hemorrhagic shock, but are difficult to standardize and vary based on the provider's skill and experience.[15]

Guyette and colleagues[16] hypothesized that in-flight measures of serum lactate and StO_2 VOT would identify shock trauma subjects in need of LSI,[17] and studied 400 transported trauma patients with lactate sampling and 194 patients also with StO_2 VOT. The aim of the study was to discover whether the StO_2 measurement, including a VOT, and spot measures of serum lactate were feasible in the prehospital air transport environment and useful to predict in-hospital death and ICU admission. Patients with prehospital lactate levels greater than 4 mmol/dL had greater need for emergent operation, intubation, and vasopressors. This association persisted after adjustment for age, Glasgow Coma Score, and initial vital signs. Not surprisingly, they did not find differences in baseline StO_2 between survivors, nonsurvivors, and patients admitted to the ICU. However, they found significant differences in DeOx and ReOx slopes between survivors and nonsurvivors, and between patients who needed ICU admission and those who did not. The StO_2VOT DeOx slopes were predictive of the need for LSI, whereas a delayed ReOx slope was predictive of mortality (**Table 1**). Furthermore, only 1 of the 5 patient deaths in their sample had prehospital vital signs that would have met the protocolized criteria for resuscitation (heart rate >120 beats/min, systolic blood pressure <90 mm Hg). Of note, serum lactate alone was no better than lowest systolic pressure in predicting those in need of LSI or death, but if the baseline serum lactate was greater than 1.7 mmol/dL the ReOx slope was 100% specific for the need of LSI. This study shows the usefulness of the microcirculation dynamic assessment in the early stages of the trauma injury, when the cardiovascular insufficiency is not suspected based solely on macrocirculatory indices.

Thus, using a functional hemodynamic monitoring approach, measures of StO_2 may provide the possibility to start the appropriate treatment earlier and decide the in-hospital disposition. These data collectively document that the measure of readily available physiologic variables, when coupled to functional hemodynamic monitoring principles (eg, VOT), predict clinically relevant physiologic states and the subsequent need for LSI.

Although the focus thus far has been on StO_2 and its changes during a VOT, other potential functional hemodynamic monitoring applications must exist, and should be useful in identifying impeding cardiovascular instability and its response to therapy.

Table 1
Tissue oximetry (Sto₂) in conjunction with a vascular occlusive test (VOT) predicts death and the need for life-saving interventions (LSI)

Variable	All Patients (n = 194)	LSI (n = 61)	No LSI (n = 133)	P
Prehospital physiology				
Highest heart rate, beats/min	98 ± 19	100 ± 19	97 ± 19	.34
Lowest systolic blood pressure	120 ± 13	119 ± 17	121 ± 10	.94
Highest respiratory rate, cycles/min	17 ± 2	18 ± 3	17 ± 2	.25
Glasgow Coma Score <15, n (%)	52 (27)	25 (41)	27 (20)	.003
Sto₂ parameters				
Deoxygenation slope, %/s	0.15 (0.1–0.2)	0.13 (0.1–0.17)	0.17 (0.11–0.21)	.007
Reoxygenation slope, %/s	2.1 (1.1–3.5)	1.9 (0.9–2.8)	2.3 (0.9–2.8)	.13
Baseline, %	80 (74–86)	80 (74–84)	80 (86–74)	.9
Prehospital serum lactate, mmol/L	2 (1.2–2.9)	2.2 (3.1–1.4)	1.8 (1.2–2.6)	.02

Variable	All Patients (n = 194)	In-Hospital Death (n = 6)	Alive at Discharge (n = 188)	P
Prehospital physiology				
Highest heart rate, beats/min	98 ± 19	94 ± 15	98 ± 19	.7
Lowest systolic blood pressure	120 ± 13	123 ± 28	120 ± 12	.3
Highest respiratory rate, cycles/min	17 ± 2	17 ± 2	17 ± 2	.9
Glasgow Coma Score <15, n (%)	53 (27)	4 (67)	49 (26)	.03
Sto₂ parameters				
Deoxygenation slope, %/s	0.15 (0.1–0.2)	0.11 (0.07–0.16)	0.15 (0.11–0.2)	.2
Reoxygenation slope, %/s	2.1 (1.1–3.5)	0.86 (0.7–0.9)	2.2 (1.3–3.5)	.005
Baseline, %	80 (74–86)	77 (68–82)	80 (74–86)	.3
Prehospital serum lactate, mmol/L	2 (1.2–2.9)	3.3 (2.4–3.8)	2 (1.2–2.9)	.08

However, a fundamental aspect of these novel monitoring devices will probably be their noninvasive nature, allowing widespread use with minimal risk, continuous in their measures, allowing trending of state, and metabolic in their orientation, because assessment of tissue wellness and metabolic status is central to defining the severity of circulatory shock.

PREDICTING VOLUME RESPONSIVENESS

A fundamental aspect of the initial resuscitation of a patient in circulatory shock is to restore MAP and global blood flow as soon as possible to minimize tissue hypoperfusion, organ injury, and subsequent inflammatory responses. Given the caveat in traumatic injury of acquiring surgical control of large vascular injuries before large volume resuscitation, all other forms of resuscitation presume a hypovolemic intravascular state in need of immediate fluid resuscitation. Clearly for the resuscitated patient presenting to the emergency department (ED) after a prolonged and progressive deterioration from slow hemorrhage, severe diarrhea, and infection, profound hypovolemia is almost universally present and requires intravascular fluid repletion. However, many patients present with preexisting cardiovascular conditions, such as heart failure, chronic obstructive pulmonary disease, diabetes, and essential hypertension, all of which limit the ability of fluid resuscitation to universally augment cardiac output. Similarly, patients already hospitalized who acutely decompensate from either occult bleed or sepsis may not present in a state of absolute hypovolemia.

Thus, it is not surprising that Michard and Teboul,[18] when reviewing all the reported studies giving fluids as the initial management of circulatory shock, found that half of the patients did not increase either cardiac output or blood pressure. Michard and Teboul refer to those patients who when in shock who do not respond favorably to an initial fluid bolus as preload nonresponders. These data suggest that as many as half of all hemodynamically unstable patients are not preload responsive, and that the blind use of fluid resuscitation as the initial management of all patients presenting in circulatory shock will be ineffective half of the time. Furthermore, fluid resuscitation has adverse effects, such a venous pressure overload promoting pulmonary and peripheral edema, acute cor pulmonale, and cerebral edema. Therefore, using clinically reliable parameters that identify patients who will respond to volume expansion helps to avoid potential harm to nonresponders of inappropriate fluid resuscitation.

Because a primary resuscitation question when addressing management of the hemodynamically unstable patient is whether patients will increase their cardiac output in response to intravascular volume infusion, knowing the volume responsiveness state is clinically important. Volume responsiveness has been arbitrarily defined as a cardiac output of 15% or greater in response to a 500-mL bolus fluid challenge. Although the presence of fluid responsiveness in a subject does not equate to the need to give fluids, it does define that if fluids are infused the cardiac output will increase.

Static Preload Measures Do Not Predict Preload Responsiveness

Cardiac preload is the maximum degree of myocardial fiber stretch or tension before ventricular contraction. When fibers are part of the ventricular wall they form hoops, such that ventricular end-diastolic volume (EDV) is usually proportional to fiber stretch. Thus, ventricular EDV is usually used as a measure of preload. Measures of ventricular filling pressures estimate which are presumed to reflect ventricular preload. Based on this knowledge, bedside clinicians seek surrogate measures of preload to guide resuscitation therapies. Unfortunately, this left ventricular (LV) volume-stretch relationship is commonly altered by myocardial ischemia and ventricular interdependence. In both cases LV diastolic compliance decreases, such that for the same EDV, as diastolic compliance decreases the wall stretch must increase. For this reason changes in LV stroke volume, as a surrogate for changes in LV preload, become unreliable during spontaneous breathing, when dynamic indices of volume responsiveness remain predictive (see later discussion).

Common clinical teaching dictates that static hemodynamic measures, such as central venous pressure (CVP), as an estimate of right ventricular (RV) filling, and pulmonary artery occlusion pressure (Ppao), as an estimate of LV filling, can be used to predict fluid responsiveness. The argument states that if CVP or Ppao are low the subject will be volume responsive, and if either is elevated the subject will not be volume responsive. However, this presumption has never been rigorously validated and, indeed, is probably incorrect over the range of pressures commonly seen in critically ill patients. Recent clinical trials and large meta-analyses of pooled studies show that static measures of either RV or LV preload do not identify those patients who will increase their cardiac output in response to fluid loading.[19–24] The reasons for this lack of clinical utility may include errors in measurement, lack of physiologic rationale, and misinterpretation of the meaning of the measures themselves. Because mechanical ventilation and spontaneous breathing often influence static measures made at the bedside differently and the physiologic interactions between heart and lung vary between these 2 forms of breathing, each are explored separately.

Estimates of preload during positive-pressure ventilation

Mechanical ventilation has a significant effect on cardiovascular function, which depends on the baseline contractility and intravascular volume status, chest wall and lung compliance, tidal volume, and ventilatory pattern.[25] Of importance, positive-pressure breathing cyclically increases in intrathoracic pressure (ITP) by forcing the expanding lungs to passively expand the chest wall. This expansion causes CVP to increase proportionally. Because CVP is the back pressure to systemic venous return to the heart, these cyclic increases in CVP cause reciprocal cyclic decreases in venous return. End-expiratory CVP is often taken as an estimate of the intravascular state. A low CVP (<8 mm Hg) is presumed to reflect a low circulating blood volume, and a high CVP an expanded blood volume.[26,27] Regrettably, neither CVP nor Ppao predict a patient's response to fluid challenges.[28–30] By meta-analysis CVP was found to have a very poor correlation with subsequent increases in cardiac output in response to a fluid challenge ($r = 0.18$), with no discriminating power.[31]

Nevertheless, CVP does have usefulness in predicting if increasing the level of positive end-expiratory pressure (PEEP) will result in a decrease in cardiac output. Jellinek and colleagues[32] examined the relationship between baseline CVP and the subsequent change in cardiac output in response to a 10-cm H_2O increase in PEEP from 0 to 10, 10 to 20, and 20 to 30 cm H_2O in 22 consecutive ventilator-dependent patients with acute respiratory distress syndrome. At all times, if the initial CVP was 8 mm Hg or less the cardiac output invariably decreased, whereas the change in cardiac output if CVP was greater than 8 mm Hg was not predictable. Accordingly, identifying ventilator-dependent patients with a low CVP ($\leq$8 mm Hg) defines a subgroup of critically ill patients at risk for decreasing cardiac output if PEEP levels are increased.

CVP can be estimated noninvasively by measuring inferior vena cava (IVC) diameter by ultrasonographic techniques using the subxiphoid window. IVC diameters less than 12 mm were predictive of volume response while values greater than 20 mm predicted nonresponders, with values in the middle not predictive at all.[20] Within this context, respiratory changes in IVC diameter may be helpful in predicting fluid response in mechanically ventilated patients as a functional hemodynamic monitoring approach. In a study of septic patients, inspiration-associated IVC diameter decreases greater than 50% correlated with a CVP of less than 8 mm Hg ($r = 0.74$).[33] Because CVP less than 8 mm Hg defines the subset of patients who will decrease their cardiac output in response to increasing PEEP, this finding is clinically relevant.

Similarly, cardiac ultrasonography can be used to identify the presence or absence of tricuspid regurgitant jets. The greater the degree of tricuspid regurgitation, the higher the estimated pulmonary artery pressure, although this measure can be inaccurate at higher pulmonary arterial pressures.

Another static measure of preload is the global EDV index (GEDVi), the summed volume of all 4 chambers of the heart, estimated by pulmonary artery to transthoracic indicator dilution transit-time differences. Not surprisingly, 80% of volume responders have GEDVi of less than 600 mL/m^2, whereas only 30% of patients with a GEDVi greater than 800 mL/m^2 are volume responders.[34] However, like IVC diameter ranges, GEDVi in the intermediate range between these 2 extremes does not distinguish volume responders from nonresponders. Theoretically, RV EDV should be a good measure of preload. Nevertheless, resuscitation efforts adding measures of GEDVi to their resuscitation algorithms allowed caregivers to choose between volume, red cell transfusion, and vasopressors in the management of critically ill patients.[35] Therefore, the use of GEDVi is not without value when used within a treatment algorithm. Another static measure obtained from the pulmonary artery thermodilution technique is the RV EDV index. Similar to the GEDVi data, RV EDV values less than 90 mL/m^2 predict volume responders while RV EDV values greater than 140 mL/m^2 predict volume nonresponders, whereas intermediate RV EDV values do not distinguish volume responders from nonresponders.[36]

Transthoracic and transesophageal echocardiography can reliably measure ventricular end-diastolic area. However, measures of end-diastolic area are also poor predictors of volume response. Nonetheless, these measures have a one-way decimatory value. If the ratio of RV end-diastolic area to LV end-diastolic area is 1 or higher, such patients are presumed to have cor pulmonale, a condition for which volume resuscitation is a contraindication even in the setting of circulatory shock, because as the right ventricle dilates further with volume loading the LV EDV progressively decreases, further worsening the state of low-output shock.[37]

Estimates of preload during spontaneous breathing

Static estimates of preload are not much better at predicting volume responsiveness during spontaneous ventilation. In general, as with positive-pressure ventilation, they are predictive at the extremes of very low/small and very high/large measures, but not predictive over a range normally seen in most critically ill patients at the start of resuscitation. Most studies primarily report on patients requiring mechanical ventilation, owing to the nature of critical illness and the cohort routinely instrumented with intravascular catheter. However, 2 studies of critically ill patients included a small subset of nonventilated patients.[38,39] Both showed, not surprisingly, that a lower initial CVP was more common in volume responders than in nonresponders. Although the CVP measures in these studies varied and the sample sizes were small, a low CVP (<5 mm Hg) identified volume responders.

The predictive value of Ppao in spontaneously breathing patients has, in general, not been described, but when reported is very poor.[40] However, one study in which 6% of the study population were spontaneously breathing patients reported that patients with a low baseline Ppao (<10 mm Hg) were volume responsive.[38] Because the use of a pulmonary artery catheter is uncommon in spontaneously breathing patients, this observation is of little practical relevance.

Using echocardiography to estimate RV and LV end-diastolic area as surrogates for EDV, 2 studies examined the relation between RV end-diastolic index (RVEDVi) and volume responsiveness. The findings mirrored those for GEDVi and RV EDV already mentioned. Subjects with increased RVEDVi (>140 mL/m^2) were not volume responsive, whereas those with reduced RVEDVi (<90 mL/m^2) were volume respon-sive. Again, patients with RVEDVi between these two extremes displayed no value of RVEDVi in predicting volume responsiveness.[36,41] Similarly to the lack of discrimi-nation using Ppao to identify volume responsiveness, LV end-diastolic area also did not discriminate between volume responders and nonresponders.[42]

Dynamic Parameters Predict Preload Responsiveness

Dynamic changes in hemodynamic variables, such as ventilation-induced changes in CVP, arterial pulse pressure, LV stroke volume, and both IVC and superior vena cava (SVC) diameter have been shown to be highly predictive of volume responsiveness in a variety of clinical scenarios. The principle behind the expression of these dynamic vari-ables is the effect of positive pressure and spontaneous ventilation on systemic venous return and, subsequently, LV output. The author has described these interac-tions in great detail elsewhere.[25] In essence, cyclic increases in ITP induced by positive-pressure breathing lung expansion also increase CVP. Because CVP is the back pressure to blood flowing back to the right ventricle from the body, referred to as venous return, if the upstream pressure does not also change then with every positive-pressure inspiration, venous return will phasically decrease. If both ventricles are volume responsive then eventually LV stroke volume must also vary, the magni-tude of this variation reflecting the degree of volume responsiveness.

Dynamic parameters in mechanically ventilated patients

Many studies have validated the usefulness of dynamic changes in arterial pulse pres-sure and LV stroke volume during positive-pressure breathing to predict with a high degree of accuracy whether a patient is going to increase cardiac output, MAP, or both in response to the volume infusion. Some of the most commonly used functional hemodynamic monitoring methods are those based on beat-to-beat changes in LV output during positive-pressure ventilation, such as pulse pressure variation (PPV) and stroke volume variation (SVV). The physiologic basis for this predictive accuracy has been well described previously.[43] In brief, during the inspiratory phase of positive-pressure ventilation, ITP increases passively, increasing right atrial pressure and causing venous return to decrease, thus decreasing RV output, and, after 2 or 3 heart beats, LV output if both ventricles are volume responsive.[43] Thus in preload-dependent patients, cyclic changes in LV stroke volume and its coupled arterial pulse pressure will be seen, the magnitude of the changes being proportional to volume responsiveness (**Fig. 2**).

However, there are many potential complicating processes that can lead to either false positives or false negatives when either PPV or SVV are measured. Understand-ing the physiologic basis for the generation of PPV and SVV thus aids in minimizing errors in their interpretation. The positive-pressure breath generated by mechanical ventilation causes cyclic increases in ITP, which simultaneously increase CVP, the back pressure to venous return. This process causes RV filling to immediately decrease because venous return to the right ventricle transiently decreases. Thus, if the right ventricle is volume responsive, RV stroke volume will also decrease on the next beat. After 2 to 3 beats this decreased pulmonary arterial inflow reaches the left ventricle, decreasing LV EDV. If the left ventricle is volume responsive, this decreased LV flow will result in a decreased LV stroke volume. Because it takes about 3 beats for the decreased RV flow to cause a decreased LV flow, the observed decreased LV stroke volume seen during positive-pressure ventilation usually occurs at the start of expiration. Thus, if both ventricles are preload responsive, positive-pressure breaths will induce dynamic changes in LV stroke volume. Because the

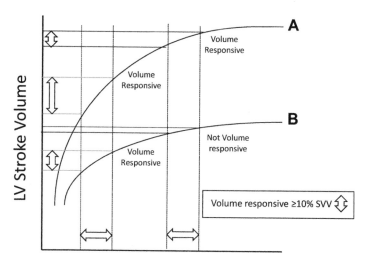

LV End-Diastolic Volume

Fig. 2. Stylized display of 2 different Frank-Starling curves showing the relation between left ventricular (LV) stroke volume and LV end-diastolic volume. If positive-pressure ventilation alters LV end-diastolic volume across a range of LV end-diastolic volumes, then LV stroke volume will also vary according to where on the Frank-Starling curve the subject is. At low levels of LV end-diastolic volume the LV stroke volume variability, quantified as stroke volume variation (SVV), will be greater than on the flatter portions of the curves. Thus, by assessing SVV for an appropriate degree of LV end-diastolic volume changes, one can reliably define where on the Frank-Starling relationship the patient is predicting subsequent change in LV stroke volume in response to increases in LV end-diastolic volume.

primary determinant of arterial pulse pressure (the increase from diastolic to systolic pressure) is stroke volume from one heart beat to the next, changes in arterial pulse pressure will also follow changes in LV stroke volume. Michard and colleagues[43] quantified the arterial PPV and the ratio of the difference between the maximal and the minimal pulse pressure over 3 breaths and the mean pulse pressure over those same breaths, reported as a percentage. These investigators demonstrated that the greater the PPV, the more the subject was volume responsive. SVV is similarly quantified as the ratio of difference between the largest and smallest LV stroke volumes to the mean LV stroke volume averaged over 3 to 5 breaths (**Fig. 3**).

Newer arterial waveform monitoring devices estimate LV stroke volume on a beat-to-beat basis, allowing continuous reporting of both PPV and SVV. Commercially available devices include PiCCO (Pulsion Medical, Feldkirchen, Germany), LiDCO (LiDCO Ltd, London, UK), Vigileo, FloTrac (Edwards Lifesciences, Irvine, CA), Most-Care (Vyetech Health, Padua, Italy), and NICOM (Cheetah Medical, Tel-Aviv, Israel), among others. The associated SVV and PPV are quantified in various ways depending on whether these are measured by minimally invasive cardiac output monitors (eg, PiCCO, LiDCO, FloTrac) or by direct examination of the pressure or flow profiles. In general, both are defined as the ratio of the maximal minus the minimal values to the mean values, usually averaged over 3 or more breaths, although one device (Flo-Trac) estimates SVV as the standard deviation of the pressure power signal to the mean power. Many commercially available minimally invasive hemodynamic monitoring devices can estimate LV stroke volume from the arterial pressure profile, giving similar SVV measures.

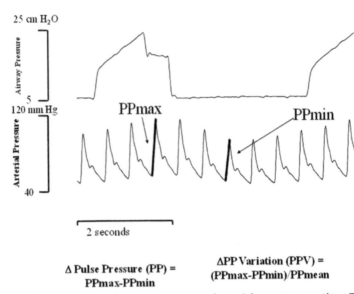

Fig. 3. A strip chart recording of airway pressure and arterial pressure over time. The ratio of the difference (Δ) between the maximal arterial pulse pressure (diastole to systole) (PPmax) and the minimal arterial pulse pressure (PPmin) to the mean pulse pressure (PPmean) defines pulse pressure variation (PPV).

Several clinical trials have documented that an SVV greater than 10% or a PPV greater than 13% to 15% on a tidal volume of 8 mL/kg or greater is highly predictive of volume responsiveness.[44–46] When PPV was compared with CVP and Ppao in tracking changes in blood volume in subjects undergoing acute normovolemic hemodilution, the change in PPV was more specific than were changes in CVP or Ppao.[20] Although PPV has a strong predictive value, a recent study has demonstrated that values between 9% and 13% are inconclusive in patients undergoing general anesthesia.[47] Heijmans and colleagues[24] examined the discriminative value of SVV in comparison with static estimates of preload in predicting volume responsiveness in ICU patients after undergoing cardiac surgery, and found that SVV was a better functional marker of fluid responsiveness than either CVP or Ppao. Thus, if the clinician is concerned about excess fluid administration, targeting a higher PPV or SVV, say 20%, would markedly increase the positive predictive value of these parameters in defining preload responsiveness. Although SVV should be an accurate predictor of preload responsiveness, it is usually estimated from the arterial pulse profile, so its accuracy would be less if the algorithm used to calculate SVV is flawed or extraneous conditions arise that make the primary assumptions questionable.

Limitations to the use of dynamic parameters to assess volume responsiveness Limitations to the use of positive-pressure induced PPV and SVV to predict volume responsiveness are listed in **Box 1**. One problem with measuring PPV and SVV is that it requires the positive-pressure breath to generate a sufficient change in ITP to cause a physiologic variation in venous return. In most studies a tidal volume of 8 mL/kg was used. Thus, tidal volumes of 6 mL/kg or less or the imposition of variable spontaneous inspiratory efforts often result in false-negative PPV and SVV values.[48] Nonetheless, if one has a PPV greater than 12% on a tidal volume of 6 mL/kg, the patient is still volume responsive.[49] Moreover, all of these techniques assume a

Box 1
Causes for inaccurate interpretation of pulse pressure variation (PPV) and stroke volume variation (SVV) threshold values to define volume responsiveness

Condition	Cause of Error
PPV or SVV false positives (PPV >15% or SVV >10% but not volume responsive)	
Spontaneous ventilation	Ventricular interdependence
Acute cor pulmonale	Ventricular interdependence
Atrial fibrillation	Variable left ventricular filling time
PPV or SVV false negatives (PPV <15% or SVV <10% but volume responsive)	
Intra-abdominal hypertension	Minimal change in the driving pressure for venous return
Small tidal volumes (<8 mL/kg)	Minimal change in the driving pressure for venous return
Bronchospasm	Minimal change in the driving pressure for venous return

fixed heart rate, so in the setting of atrial fibrillation or frequent premature ventricular contractions these measures become inaccurate. In these settings, alternative approaches to PPV and SVV can be used while still using the same functional hemodynamic monitoring logic.

A major problem in using PPV or SVV is the need for a constant R-R interval (constant heart rate) so that diastolic filling time is not contributing to the preload effect of the positive-pressure breath. Thus, in patients with frequent premature ventricular contractions or atrial fibrillation, the accuracy of these parameters degrades markedly.

Another problem with the use of PPV and SVV in predicting fluid responsiveness is its false-positive rate in the setting of right heart failure. With acute cor pulmonale, positive-pressure inspiration decreases RV EDV, making the left ventricle more compliant and increasing LV EDV and LV stroke volume, even though RV failure limits fluid responsiveness. Thus, in the setting of right heart failure, PPV and SVV may be misleading. In this regard, both PPV and SVV were examined as predictors of volume responsiveness in patients with RV failure. While increases of CVP, SVV, and PPV were suggestive of RV failure, SVV and PPV failed to predict volume responsiveness in these patients.[50] Thus caution needs to be exercised in interpreting PPV and SVV in patients with RV failure.

Intra-abdominal hypertension also invalidates the use of PPV and SVV, as a patient may remain volume responsive even if the PPV is less than 15% and the SVV less than 10%, because in the setting of intra-abdominal hypertension, as the diaphragm descends during the positive-pressure breath the intra-abdominal pressure increases almost as much as the ITP, so that no decreases in pressure gradients for venous return are created.

Alternative dynamic measures to pulse-pressure variation and stroke volume variation Alternatives to PPV measures can be assessed using similar functional hemodynamic monitoring principles. Monnet and colleagues[51] examined the effect of a 15-second end-expiratory pause on the change in arterial pulse pressure to predict fluid responsiveness; they reasoned that the end-expiratory pause would allow venous return to increase, causing an increase in arterial pulse pressure in comparison with positive-pressure breathing. In 34 patients under mechanical ventilation, a 15% ± 15% arterial pulse-pressure increase correlated with a 12% ± 11% cardiac index increase.

Alternative measures to pulse pressure or left ventricular stroke volume As described earlier, ultrasonographic measures of IVC diameter reflect estimates of preload, and respiratory variations in IVC diameter also predict volume responsiveness in ventilated patients. During positive-pressure inspiration, the increased ITP transmits to the right atrium, reducing venous return and causing IVC dilation, whereas during expiration the decreased ITP increases venous return and decreases IVC diameter. Presumably the dynamic changes in IVC diameter will be greater the more volume responsive a subject is. In support of this assumption, studies in septic patients demonstrated that changes in IVC diameter greater than 12% or IVC collapsibility index of at least 18% differentiated volume responders from nonresponders.[52,53] Similarly, change in SVC diameter can be used. An SVC collapsibility index greater than 36% has sensitivity and sensitivity in identifying volume responders similar to those of the IVC collapsibility index.[50,54,55] However, SVC imaging can only reliably be done using transesophageal echocardiography. Since newer continuous transesophageal echocardiographic approaches have been introduced (hTEE, IMACOR), the use of the SVC collapsibility index has increased in popularity.[56]

Besides SVV, PPV, and IVC collapsibility index measures, there are other dynamic parameters based on the same physiologic mechanisms. Unfortunately, these other indirect measures are less predictive than SVV and PPV. These other parameters derived from arterial pressure analysis include systolic pressure variation (SPV), aortic blood flow velocity recorded via esophageal Doppler ultrasonography,[57,58] pressure wave variation by pulse oximetry, aortic flow velocity time,[59,60] and brachial flow variation time.[61] Plethysmographic wave via pulse oximetry (Pplet) is a noninvasive dynamic parameter that mirrors arterial pulse pressure. In mechanically ventilated patients, studies have shown a good correlation between PPV and Pplet.[62] In the setting of spontaneously breathing patients, however, there is a lack of agreement on the ability of Pplet to predict volume response. Because Pplet can be readily measured in any patient with a finger-pulse oximeter, the potential application of this approach needs to be further studied.

Passive leg-raising maneuver A classic method for assessing volume responsiveness in general is to note the transient effects of a passive leg-raising (PLR) maneuver on cardiac output and its surrogate markers. This approach is especially useful in identifying volume responsiveness in patients with arrhythmias and/or spontaneous breathing. The PLR maneuver is performed by passively raising both legs to an angle of 45° with respect to the bed for at least 1 minute while continuously measuring cardiac output. The PLR maneuver is equivalent to giving a 70-kg patient a transient volume bolus of 300 mL.[63] This maneuver essentially transfers blood from the lower extremities to the intrathoracic vessels, causing an increase in intrathoracic blood volume. If the subject is volume responsive, the PLR will increase cardiac output by at least 10%.[64,65] In the critically ill patient, raising the legs may cause pain and discomfort. A more gentle method of accomplishing the same effect is to rotate the bed from a semirecumbent position to a supine one and hold it there for 3 minutes. Usually patients requiring mechanical ventilation are placed in a semirecumbent position with the head of the bed elevated 30° to 45°. Thus, simply rotating the bed so that the back is supine will elevate the legs 30° to 45°. Marik and colleagues[66] showed that the change in cardiac output in response to PLR, as measured completely noninvasively using bioreactance alone[67] and when combined with Doppler ultrasonography, also predicted volume responsiveness in critically ill patients. Because this PLR maneuver is temporary, it only identifies those subjects who are volume responsive, and is not a therapy unto itself. The Pplet density change can also be used as a surrogate for arterial pulse pressure changes in response to a PLR to predict fluid response in ED subjects.[68] Unfortunately, the follow-up study 2 years later by the same ED group, using the same PLR maneuver, found no correlation between changes in Pplet during the PLR maneuver and subsequent changes in cardiac index in response to fluid challenge.[69] Thus, it is unclear as to whether Pplet can be used as a surrogate for arterial pulse pressure across volume challenge tests. Potentially, the poorer performance of the Pplet parameter in the follow-up article may have been due to their studying patients following abdominal surgery. Because of the associated increased intra-abdominal pressure altering fluid shifts, PLR maneuvers cannot accurately predict fluid responsiveness in patients with intra-abdominal hypertension.[70]

Dynamic parameters in spontaneously breathing patients

Essentially, with spontaneous inspiratory efforts the ITP decreases, owing to the opposing effects of lung parenchymal stiffness resisting expansion and chest wall/diaphragm contraction increasing thoracic compartment volume. The right atrial wall is highly compliant, so all of the decrease in ITP is transferred to the right atrial cavity, decreasing right atrial pressure or CVP. Because CVP is the back pressure to venous return, decreases in CVP will accelerate venous blood flow back to the heart during spontaneous inspiration. If the right ventricle is volume responsive, its filling pressure will increase less than the decrease in ITP. Thus CVP will decrease during spontaneous inspiration in patients who are volume responsive. If the right ventricle is not volume responsive the initial acceleration of venous return will dilate the right ventricle, increasing RV end-diastolic pressure and CVP. Such spontaneous inspiration-associated increase in CVP is called the Kussmual sign and reflects cor pulmonale or tamponade.[71] In any case, patients with a Kussmual sign are not volume responsive. The associated changes in LV EDV are not preload dependent but are due to changes in LV diastolic compliance owing to ventricular interdependence.

Dynamic changes in central venous pressure Using the dynamic changes in CVP during spontaneous ventilation, Magder and colleagues[72] predicted that those patents breathing spontaneously who displayed a decrease in CVP of greater than 1 mm Hg would be volume responsive, whereas those who did not would not be volume responsive. In 33 ICU patients, 12 of whom were breathing spontaneously, a CVP decrease greater than 1 mm Hg predicted volume responsiveness in 13 of 14 positive patients and predicted nonresponsiveness in 16 of 19 other patients.[72] Although simple, this approach is seldom used because of the inherent difficulty in identifying small changes in CVP apart from those caused by the normal cardiac cycle.

Spontaneous inspiration decreases ITP and CVP, causing venous return to accelerate, and increasing RV EDV. The sudden increase in RV EDV decreases LV diastolic compliance by the process of ventricular interdependence. Thus, for the same LV filling pressure the LV EDV decreases. Because preload is LV wall stress, not volume, if diastolic compliance decreases then for the same filling pressure LV EDV will also decrease but LV wall stress will remain constant. Thus, LV stroke volume will change even though preload has not changed. Hence during spontaneous ventilation, only right-sided changes in ventricular function assessed by dynamic swings in CVP can be presumed to reflect dynamic changes in preload,[73] whereas PPV and SVV, if present, may reflect ventricular interdependence rather than volume responsiveness.

Use of the Valsalva maneuver to assess volume responsiveness The most commonly studied dynamic parameter of volume responsiveness during spontaneous ventilation is the associated change in arterial pulse pressure and systolic pressure associated with the various phases of a Valsalva maneuver. The Valsalva maneuver is traditionally divided into 3 phases: the initial strain, the sustained strain, and the immediate release and reactive overshoot. During the initial strain of a Valsalva maneuver, airway pressure and ITP increase equally because lung volume is held constant by the occluded airway. Thus, pulmonary vascular resistance remains constant. During this first phase of the Valsalva maneuver, RV filling decreases because venous return decreases, with no immediate change in LV filling, LV stroke volume, or arterial pulse pressure. Although LV stroke volume does not change, LV peak ejection pressure increases equal to the amount of the increase in ITP.[74] Thus, systolic arterial pressure increases but pulse pressure remains constant. As the strain is sustained, both LV filling and cardiac output decrease owing to the decrease in venous return,[75] which results in the second phase. During this second phase of the Valsalva maneuver, both RV and LV output are decreased, reflected in a decreased arterial pulse pressure. However, because ITP remains elevated, MAP is also maintained. With release of the strain in phase 3 of the Valsalva maneuver, arterial pressure abruptly declines as the low LV stroke volume cannot sustain an adequate ejection pressure on its own. At the same time, however, with the release of the increased ITP venous return increases, increasing RV volume, and, through the process of ventricular interdependence, decreases LV diastolic compliance, reducing LV EDV even further. Thus, MAP rapidly decreases owing to the loss of the ITP and a lowering LV EDV. Under normal conditions a phase 4 hyperdynamic rebound occurs, increasing both peak systolic pressure and arterial pulse pressure. This arterial pressure "overshoot" identifies adequate cardiovascular reserve. Lack of an increase in pulse pressure, connoted as the "square wave" response on release, identifies those patients with impaired ventricular pump function.[76,77] Recently these phases were assessed by the associated arterial PPV across phases as opposed to across breaths, here defined as the greatest difference in arterial pulse pressure between minimal and maximal beats over the Valsalva maneuver. Using this approach, Monge Garcia and colleagues[61] found that a Valsalva PPV greater than 52% predicted a positive response to fluid administration with 91% sensitivity and 95% specificity, respectively.

Both mechanically ventilated and spontaneously breathing

One can examine the increase in arterial pulse pressure with end-expiratory pause in patients spontaneously triggering positive pressure breaths while on mechanical ventilatory support, such as pressure-support ventilation, as described earlier for positive-pressure breathing.[51] In this case, however, threshold values of 20% for both PPV and SVV are needed to be predictive of volume responsiveness.

Limitations to Predicting Volume Responsiveness

Volume responsiveness has been arbitrarily defined as an increase of 15% or greater in cardiac output as a response to a 500-mL fluid challenge. However, these cutoff values for increase in flow and volume administered are both arbitrary and misleading. Clearly the responses are linear, and the amount of volume given should be relative to the presumed effective blood volume, a value dependent on patient size, age, and sex. Similarly, some volume-responsive patients may increase their MAP more than their cardiac output, whose own increase in cardiac output may be below the threshold for measurement. Whether small increases in cardiac output in the management of patients at risk for tissue hypoperfusion reduce morbidity and mortality is not clear if, but any such treatment must be balanced by the concern for fluid overload. Thus, continuing to fluid-resuscitate patients until they are no longer volume responsive will markedly overresuscitate those patients with a normal ventricular response.

Although the presence of fluid responsiveness does not necessarily imply the need for fluid resuscitation, nor does it guarantee that if fluids are given to increase cardiac output that the increase in blood flow will reverse tissue hypoperfusion.[78] In mechanically ventilated patients, the major limitations are the inherent dependence on ventilator-induced changes in ITP large enough to change CVP. Therefore, as listed in **Box 1**, tidal volumes less than 6 mL/kg or irregular spontaneous respirations will give false-positive PPV and SVV. Furthermore, these dynamic measures rely on heart rate regularity, so arrhythmias such as atrial fibrillation can render these measures inaccurate. However, the cardiac output response to PLR will perform well in the setting of arrhythmias.[57]

Finally, defining volume responsiveness by giving small volumes of fluid is not the same as fluid resuscitation. Both small fluid bolus challenges and PLR merely document volume responsiveness. Aggressive fluid resuscitation in volume-responsive patients in shock improves outcome.[79] Thus, although it may be more efficient to use end points of fluid therapy based on the disappearance of preload responsiveness rather than static values of preload in guiding fluid therapy in critically ill patients in shock, a more reasonable approach would be to determine when resuscitation has reversed measures of organ and tissue hypoperfusion.[80]

REFERENCES

1. Pinsky MR. Functional hemodynamic monitoring: use of derived variable to diagnose and manage the critically ill. Acta Anaesthesiol Scand 2009;53(Suppl 119):9–11.
2. Pinsky MR. Hemodynamic evaluation and monitoring in the ICU. Chest 2007; 123:2020–9.
3. Georger JF, Hamzaoui O, Chaari A, et al. Restoring arterial pressure with norepinephrine improves muscle tissue oxygen saturation assessed by near-infrared spectroscopy in severely hypotensive septic patients. Intensive Care Med 2010;36:1882–9.
4. Pearse R, Dawson D, Fawcet J, et al. Early goal-directed therapy after major surgery reduces complications and duration of hospital stay. A randomised, controlled trial. Crit Care 2005;9:R687–93.
5. Pottecher J, Deruddre S, Teboul JL, et al. Both passive leg raising and intravascular volume expansion improve sublingual microcirculatory perfusion in severe sepsis and septic shock patients. Intensive Care Med 2010;36:1867–74.
6. Gomez H, Torres A, Zenker S, et al. Use of non-invasive NIRS during vascular occlusion test to assess dynamic tissue O_2 saturation response. Intensive Care Med 2008;34:1600–7.
7. Creteur J, Carollo T, Soldati G, et al. The prognostic value of muscle StO_2 in septic patients. Intensive Care Med 2007;33:1549–56.
8. De Backer D, Creteur J, Preiser JC, et al. Microvascular blood flow is altered in patients with sepsis. Am J Respir Crit Care Med 2002;166:98–104.
9. Sakr Y, Dubois MJ, De Backer D, et al. Persistent microcirculatory alterations are associated with organ failure and death in patients with septic shock. Crit Care Med 2004;34:1825–31.
10. Mesquida J, Espinal C, Graurtmoner G, et al. Prognostic implications of tissue oxygenation in human septic shock. Intensive Care Med 2012;38:592–7.
11. Guyette FX, Gomez H, Suffoletto B, et al. Prehospital dynamic tissue O_2 saturation response predicts in-hospital morality in trauma patients. J Trauma 2012;72:930–5.
12. Wo CC, Shoemaker WC, Appel PL, et al. Unreliability of blood pressure and heart rate to evaluate cardiac output in emergency resuscitation and critical illness. Crit Care Med 1993;21:218–23.

13. Holcomb JB, Niles SE, Miller CC, et al. Prehospital physiologic data and life-saving interventions in trauma patients. Mil Med 2005;170:7–13.
14. Holcomb JB, Salinas J, McManus JJ, et al. Manual vital signs reliably predict need for life-saving interventions in trauma patients. J Trauma 2005;59:821–9.
15. Porter JM, Ivatury RR. In search of the optimal end points of resuscitation in trauma patients: a review. J Trauma 1998;44:908–14.
16. Guyette FX, Suffoletto BP, Castillio JL, et al. Identification of occult shock using out-of-hospital lactate. Ann Emerg Med 2009;54:S142.
17. Castillio JL, Guyette FX, Suffoletto BP, et al. The role of prehospital lactate as a predictor of outcomes in trauma patients. J Trauma 2009;63:S138.
18. Michard F, Teboul JL. Predicting fluid responsiveness in ICU patients: a critical analysis of the evidence. Chest 2002;121:2000–8.
19. Sabatier C, Monge I, Maynar J, et al. Assessment of cardiovascular preload and response to volume expansion. Med Intensiva 2012;36:45–55.
20. Sant'Ana AJ, Otsuki DA, Noel-Morgan J, et al. Use of pulse pressure variation to estimate changes in preload during experimental acute normovolemic hemodilution. Minerva Anestesiol 2012;78:426–33.
21. Pereira de Souza Neto E, Grousson S, Duflo F, et al. Predicting fluid responsiveness in mechanically ventilated children under general anaesthesia using dynamic parameters and transthoracic echocardiography. Br J Anaesth 2011; 106:856–64.
22. Eichhorn V, Trepte C, Richter HP, et al. Respiratory systolic variation test in acutely impaired cardiac function for predicting volume responsiveness in pigs. Br J Anaesth 2011;106:659–64.
23. Maguire S, Rinehart J, Vakharia S, et al. Technical communication: respiratory variation in pulse pressure and plethysmographic waveforms: intraoperative applicability in a North American academic center. Anesth Analg 2011;112:94–6.
24. Heijmans JH, Ganushak YM, Theunissen MS, et al. Predictors of cardiac responsiveness to fluid therapy after cardiac surgery. Acta Anaesthesiol Belg 2010;61:151–8.
25. Pinsky MR. Heart-lung interactions during mechanical ventilation. In: Bakker J, editor. Cardiopulmonary monitoring. Curr Opin Crit Care 2012;18:256–60.
26. Pinsky MR. The hemodynamic consequences of mechanical ventilation: an evolving story. Intensive Care Med 1997;23:493–503.
27. Bendjelid K, Romand JA. Fluid responsiveness in mechanically ventilated patients: a review of indices used in intensive care. Intensive Care Med 2003;29: 352–60.
28. Kumar A, Anel R, Bunnell E, et al. Pulmonary artery occlusion pressure and central venous pressure fail to predict ventricular filling volume, cardiac performance, or the response to volume infusion in normal subjects. Crit Care Med 2004;32:691–9.
29. Malbrain ML. Is it wise not to think about intraabdominal hypertension in the ICU? Curr Opin Crit Care 2004;10:132–45.
30. Pinsky MR. Clinical significance of pulmonary artery occlusion pressure. Intensive Care Med 2003;29:175–8.
31. Marik PE, Baram M, Vahid B. Does central venous pressure predict fluid responsiveness? A systematic review of the literature and the tale of seven mares. Chest 2008;134:172–8.
32. Jellinek H, Krafft P, Fitzgerald RD, et al. Right atrial pressure predicts hemodynamic response to apneic positive airway pressure. Crit Care Med 2000;28: 672–8.

33. Nagdev AD, Merchant RC, Tirado-Gonzalez A, et al. Emergency department bedside ultrasonographic measurement of the caval index for noninvasive determination of low central venous pressure. Ann Emerg Med 2010;55: 290–5.
34. Michard F, Alaya S, Zarka V, et al. Global end-diastolic volume as an indicator of cardiac preload in patients with septic shock. Chest 2003;124:1900–10.
35. Yu M, Pei K, Moran S, et al. A prospective randomized trial using blood volume analysis in addition to pulmonary artery catheter compared with pulmonary artery catheter alone, to guide shock resuscitation in critically ill surgical patients. Shock 2011;35:220–8.
36. Reuse C, Vincent JL, Pinsky MR. Measurements of right ventricular volumes during fluid challenge. Chest 1990;98:1450–4.
37. Coudray A, Romand JA, Treggiari M, et al. Fluid responsiveness in spontaneously breathing patients: a review of indexes used in intensive care. Crit Care Med 2005;33:2757–62.
38. Wagner JG, Leatherman JW. Right ventricular end-diastolic volume as a predictor of the hemodynamic response to a fluid challenge. Chest 1998;113:1048–54.
39. Schneider AJ, Teule GJ, Groeneveld AB, et al. Biventricular performance during volume loading in patients with early septic shock, with emphasis on the right ventricle: a combined hemodynamic and radionuclide study. Am Heart J 1988;116:103–12.
40. Calvin JE, Driedger AA, Sibbald WJ. The hemodynamic effect of rapid fluid infusion in critically ill patients. Surgery 1981;90:61–76.
41. Diebel LN, Wilson RF, Tagett MG, et al. End-diastolic volume. A better indicator of preload in the critically ill. Arch Surg 1992;127:817–21.
42. Lamia B, Ochagavia A, Monnet X, et al. Echocardiographic prediction of volume responsiveness in critically ill patients with spontaneously breathing activity. Intensive Care Med 2007;33:1125–32.
43. Michard F, Boussat S, Chemla D, et al. Relation between respiratory changes in arterial pulse pressure and fluid responsiveness in septic patients with acute circulatory failure. Am J Respir Crit Care Med 2000;162:134–8.
44. Berkenstadt H, Margalit N, Hadani M, et al. Stroke volume variation as a predictor of fluid responsiveness in patients undergoing brain surgery. Anesth Analg 2001;92:984–9.
45. Montenij LJ, de Waal EE, Buhre WF. Arterial waveform analysis in anesthesia and critical care. Curr Opin Anaesthesiol 2011;24:651–6.
46. Michard F. Changes in arterial pressure during mechanical ventilation. Anesthesiology 2005;103:419–28.
47. Cannesson M, Le Manach Y, Hofer CK, et al. Assessing the diagnostic accuracy of pulse pressure variations for the prediction of fluid responsiveness: a "gray zone" approach. Anesthesiology 2011;115:231–41.
48. DeBacker D, Heenen S, Piagenrelli M, et al. Pulse pressure variations to predict fluid responsiveness: influence of tidal volume. Intensive Care Med 2005;31: 517–23.
49. Huang CC, Fu JY, Hu HV, et al. Prediction of fluid responsiveness in acute respiratory distress syndrome patients ventilated with low tidal volume and high positive end-expiratory pressure. Crit Care Med 2008;36:2810–6.
50. Richter HP, Petersen C, Goetz AE, et al. Detection of right ventricular insufficiency and guidance of volume therapy are facilitated by simultaneous monitoring of static and functional preload parameters. J Cardiothorac Vasc Anesth 2011;25:1051–5.

51. Monnet X, Osman D, Ridel C, et al. Predicting volume responsiveness by using the end-expiratory occlusion in mechanically ventilated intensive care unit patients. Crit Care Med 2009;37:951–6.
52. Barbier C, Loubieres Y, Schmit C, et al. Respiratory changes in inferior vena cava diameter are helpful in predicting fluid responsiveness in ventilated septic patients. Intensive Care Med 2004;30:1740–6.
53. Feissel M, Michard F, Faller JP, et al. The respiratory variation in inferior vena cava diameter as a guide to fluid therapy. Intensive Care Med 2004;30:1834–7.
54. Jardin F, Vieillard-Baron A. Ultrasonographic examination of the venae cavae. Intensive Care Med 2006;32:203–6.
55. Vieillard-Baron A, Chergui K, Rabiller A, et al. Superior vena caval collapsibility as a gauge of volume status in ventilated septic patients. Intensive Care Med 2004;30:1734–9.
56. Vieillard-Baron A, Slama M, Mayo P, et al. A pilot study on safety and clinical utility of a single-use 72-hour indwelling transesophageal echocardiographic probe. Intensive Care Med 2013;39:629–35.
57. Monnet X, Rienzo M, Osman D, et al. Esophageal Doppler monitoring predicts fluid responsiveness in critically ill ventilated patients. Intensive Care Med 2005; 31:1195–201.
58. Slama M, Masson H, Teboul JL, et al. Monitoring of respiratory variations of aortic blood flow velocity using esophageal Doppler. Intensive Care Med 2004;30:1182–7.
59. Slama M, Masson H, Teboul JL, et al. Respiratory variations of aortic VTI: a new index of hypovolemia and fluid responsiveness. Am J Physiol 2002;283: H1729–33.
60. Feissel M, Michard F, Mangin I, et al. Respiratory changes in aortic blood velocity as an indicator of fluid responsiveness in ventilated patients with septic shock. Chest 2001;119:867–73.
61. Monge Garcia MI, Gil Cano A, Diaz Monrove JC. Arterial pressure changes during the Valsalva maneuver to predict fluid responsiveness in spontaneously breathing patients. Intensive Care Med 2009;35:77–84.
62. Cannesson M, Desebbe O, Rosamek P, et al. Pleth variability index to monitor the respiratory variations in the pulse oximeter plethysmographic waveform amplitude and predict fluid responsiveness in the operating theatre. Br J Anaesth 2008;101:200–6.
63. Monnet X, Teboul JL. Passive leg raising. In: Pinsky MR, Brochard L, Mancebo J, et al, editors. Applied physiology in intensive care medicine 2: physiologic reviews and editorial. Spring-Verlag Berlin; 2012. p. 55–61.
64. Jabot J, Teboul JL, Richard C, et al. Passive leg raising for predicting fluid responsiveness: importance of the postural change. Intensive Care Med 2009;35:85–90.
65. Cavallaro F, Sandroni C, Marano C, et al. Diagnostic accuracy of passive leg raising for prediction of fluid responsiveness in adults: systematic review and meta-analysis of clinical studies. Intensive Care Med 2010;36:1475–83.
66. Marik PE, Levitov A, Young A, et al. The use of bioreactance and carotid Doppler to determine volume responsiveness and blood flow redistribution following passive leg raising in hemodynamically unstable patients. Chest 2013;143: 364–70.
67. Benomar B, Ouattara A, Estagnasie P, et al. Fluid responsiveness predicted by noninvasive Bioreactance-based passive leg raise test. Intensive Care Med 2010;36:1875–81.

68. Delerme S, Renault R, Le Manach Y, et al. Variations in pulse oximetry plethysmographic waveform amplitude induced by passive leg raising in spontaneously breathing volunteers. Am J Emerg Med 2007;25:637–42.

69. Delerme S, Castro S, Freund Y, et al. Relation between pulse oximetry plethysmographic waveform amplitude induced by passive leg raising and cardiac index in spontaneously breathing subjects. Am J Emerg Med 2010;28:505–10.

70. Mahjoub Y, Touzeau J, Airapetian N, et al. The passive leg-raising maneuver cannot accurately predict fluid responsiveness in patients with intra-abdominal hypertension. Crit Care Med 2010;38:1824–9.

71. Dell'Italia LJ, Starling MR, O'Rourke RA. Physical examination for exclusion of hemodynamically important right ventricular infarction. Ann Intern Med 1983; 99:608–11.

72. Magder S, Georgiadis G, Cheong T. Respiratory variations in right atrial pressure predict the response to fluid challenge. J Crit Care 1992;7:76–85.

73. Clyne C, Alpert JS, Benotti JR. Interdependence of the left and right ventricles in health and disease. Am Heart J 1989;117:16–73.

74. Fletcher EC, Proctor M, Yu J, et al. Pulmonary edema develops after recurrent obstructive apneas. Am J Respir Crit Care Med 1999;160:1688–96.

75. Sharpey-Schaffer EP. Effects of Valsalva maneuver on the normal and failing circulation. Br Med J 1955;1:693–9.

76. Zema MJ, Restivo B, Sos T, et al. Left ventricular dysfunction-bedside Valsalva maneuver. Heart 1980;44:560–9.

77. Zema MJ, Masters AP, Margouleff D. Dyspnea: the heart or the lungs? Differentiation at the bedside by the use of a simple Valsalva maneuver. Chest 1984;85: 59–64.

78. Garcia X, Pinsky MR. Clinical applicability of functional hemodynamic monitoring. Ann Intensive Care 2011;1:35.

79. Dellinger RP, Levy MM, Carlet JM, et al. Surviving sepsis campaign: international guidelines for management of severe sepsis and septic shock. Crit Care Med 2008;36:296–327.

80. Vincent JL, DeBacker D. Circulatory shock. N Engl J Med 2013;369:1726–33.

Defining Goals of Resuscitation in the Critically Ill Patient

Alexandre Joosten, MD[a,b], Brenton Alexander, BS[a],
Maxime Cannesson, MD, PhD[a,*]

KEYWORDS

- Oxygen delivery • Oxygen consumption • Goal-directed fluid therapy
- Cardiac output optimization

KEY POINTS

- Understand the goals of resuscitation in the critically ill patient using target perfusion pressures, flows, and oxygen delivery/consumption targets for specific patient groups based on disease process.
- Understand the difference in management approaches for intraoperative and intensive care unit critically ill patients.
- Understand the major physiologic variables used for defining cardiopulmonary medicine.
- Understand the major physiologic endpoints for assessment of adequate fluid optimization.
- Be familiar with the concept of goal-directed fluid therapy and understand the importance of such a therapeutic protocol in the future of fluid management.

INTRODUCTION

As stated by Arthur Guyton in his *Textbook of Medical Physiology*:

> *The function of the circulation is to service the needs of the body tissues, to transport nutrients to the body tissues, to transport waste products away, to conduct hormones from one part of the body to another, and, in general, to maintain an*

Financial Interest: These authors have identified no professional or financial affiliations for themselves or their spouse/partner: A. Joosten, B. Alexander. Dr M. Cannesson has identified the following professional or financial affiliations for himself or his spouse/partner: Dr M. Cannesson is a consultant for Edwards Lifesciences, LidCO, Massimo, Deltex and is part founder and shareholder in Sironis Inc.
[a] Department of Anesthesiology and Perioperative Care, University of California, Irvine, 101 The City Drive South, Orange, CA 92868, USA; [b] Department of Anesthesiology and Critical Care, Erasme University Hospital, Free University of Brussels, 808 Lennick Road, Brussels 1070, Belgium
* Corresponding author.
E-mail address: mcanness@uci.edu

Crit Care Clin 31 (2015) 113–132
http://dx.doi.org/10.1016/j.ccc.2014.08.006
0749-0704/15/$ – see front matter © 2015 Elsevier Inc. All rights reserved.

appropriate environment in all the tissue fluids of the body for optimal survival and function of the cells. To be achieved, this goal requires two physiological objectives:

Adequate perfusion pressure in order to force blood into the capillaries of all organs.

Adequate cardiac output to deliver oxygen and substrates, and to remove carbon dioxide and other metabolic products.[1,2]

In daily practice, we are often confronted by critically ill patients in different settings that require hemodynamic optimization to restore or maintain sufficient tissue perfusion. Hemodynamic optimization is specific to each "patient population" and the critically ill patient in the intensive care unit (ICU) is not the same as the surgical patient undergoing high-risk surgery. Optimal perfusion therefore depends on patient-specific disease processes. For example, in the ICU, clinicians have to deal with very unstable patients with their main objective being the restoration of adequate circulation through careful correction of the blood flow and resulting oxygen delivery (Do_2). On the other hand, the major concern of the anesthetist in the perioperative period is to (1) optimize the patient's volemic status by maximizing Do_2 through "well-defined" goals using flow-related hemodynamic parameters and (2) avoid any impairment in Do_2 or cardiac output (CO). Regardless of setting, critically ill patients often present with hypovolemia, and volume expansion is one of the most frequent clinical interventions performed in daily practice. It is commonly the first treatment for hemodynamic resuscitation because it can increase Do_2 to the tissues, through increasing left ventricular stroke volume (SV) and CO.

As with most critical interventions, an appropriate end point for such fluid therapy has been widely researched and is constantly adapting to new technologies and outcome investigations. This concept of targeting predefined goals of resuscitation in critically ill patient is not novel. Goal-directed therapy (GDT) has come to encompass the concept of using established targets of continuous blood flow and/or tissue oxygenation to guide therapy (intravenous fluid and/or inotropes). This strategy is becoming the standard of care in the ICU and in the operating rooms. However, despite studies suggesting that this approach is beneficial, GDT is still poorly adopted in clinical practice[3,4] and, in many cases, fluids are still administered without adequate goals and monitoring to guide volume therapy. This can lead to adverse clinical outcomes related to hypovolemia or hypervolemia (**Table 1**). Both risks can potentially lead to a decrease in Do_2 to the tissues and to an increase in postoperative morbidity (**Fig. 1**).[5] Therefore, the optimization of the patient's hemodynamics through targets of resuscitation is one of the most important goals to improving patient morbidity and mortality.

PHYSIOLOGY

In this article, the physiologic basis of Do_2, oxygen consumption (Vo_2), and their implications for the clinician are described. One of the most important questions for a clinician at the bedside of a critically ill patient must be: "Is oxygen delivery sufficient to meet the patient's cellular oxygen demand?" If the answer to this question is not confidently affirmative, a clinician risks exposing his patient to cellular ischemia, organ dysfunction, and death. Knowing the adequacy of the patient's oxygen transport balance is essential to the understanding of the pathophysiology and management of critically ill patients. Therefore, one should always keep in mind the determinants of Do_2 and consumption (**Fig. 2**).

Oxygen delivery (Do_2) is the total amount of oxygen delivered to body tissues by the heart per minute and is expressed using the following equation (HR, heart rate; Sao_2,

Table 1
Comparison between complications associated with hypervolemia and hypovolemia

Complications of Hypervolemia	Complications of Hypovolemia
Increases venous pressure resulting in loss of fluid from the intravascular to interstitial space, which can lead to pulmonary and peripheral edema impairing tissue oxygenation	Reduces effective blood circulatory volume resulting in diversion of blood flow from nonvital organs (skin, gut, kidneys) to vital organs (heart and brain)
Increases demand on cardiac function	Activates the sympathetic nervous and renin angiotensin system
Decreases tissue oxygenation with delayed wound healing	Increases inflammatory response
May cause coagulation disturbances through hemodilution	May also lead to vasopressor agent administration, which may increase hypoperfusion and ischemia[99]
Is associated with increased daily fluid balance and mortality.[100] Chappell et al also demonstrates a relationship between weight gain related to excessive fluid administration and mortality[101]	

arterial hemoglobin oxygen saturation; Hb, hemoglobin concentration; Pao_2, arterial oxygen partial pressure):

$$Do_2 \, (mL/min) = Cardiac\ output\,(CO, L/min) \times Arterial\ oxygen\ content\,(Cao_2, mL\,O_2/dL)$$

$$Do_2 \, (mL/min) = HR \times SV \times [(Sao_2 \times Hb \times 1.34) + (0.003 \times Pao_2)]$$

Increasing Do_2 is achieved through 2 different approaches: increasing CO and Cao_2. Generally, CO is more frequently manipulated by using fluids and/or inotrope agents. Conversely, Cao_2 is most commonly increased by augmenting Sao_2 and/or Hb concentration because the quantity of dissolved O_2 is low.

Oxygen consumption (Vo_2) is the volume of oxygen consumed by the tissues per minute (Cao_2; Cvo_2, venous oxygen content).

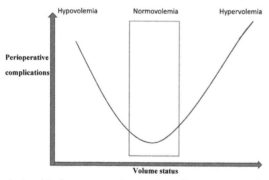

Fig. 1. The classic relationship between perioperative volume status and perioperative complications. The relationship describes a U shape with an increased risk of complication for both perioperative hypovolemia and perioperative hypervolemia, emphasizing the importance of perioperative fluid optimization.

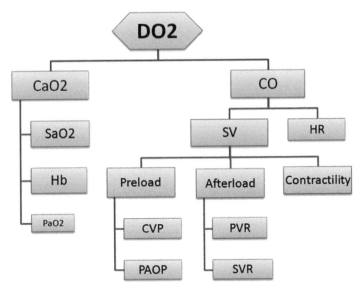

Fig. 2. Flowchart describing composition of the delivery of oxygen to tissues throughout the body. PVR, peripheric vascular resistance.

V_{O_2} (mL/min) = CO (L/min) × [Ca_{O_2} − Cv_{O_2} (mL O_2/dL)]

Oxygen demand is the amount of oxygen required by the tissues to function aerobically.

Extraction oxygen ratio (EOR) in the tissues is defined as follows:

EOR = V_{O_2}/D_{O_2}

EOR = [CO × (Ca_{O_2} − Cv_{O_2})]/[CO × (Sa_{O_2} × Hb × 1.34)]

Venous oxygen saturation (Sv_{O_2}) can then be calculated and reduced to the following formula:

Sv_{O_2} = Sa_{O_2} − (V_{O_2}/(CO × Hb × 1.34))

Any decrease in Sv_{O_2} may therefore result from a decrease in Sa_{O_2}, a decrease in CO, a decrease in hemoglobin level, or an increase in V_{O_2}. Providing that Sa_{O_2}, V_{O_2}, and hemoglobin level are in normal ranges, Sv_{O_2} can then be used as a surrogate for CO.

Also, if V_{O_2} = CO × (Ca_{O_2} − Cv_{O_2}), D_{O_2} (mL/min) = CO × [(Sa_{O_2} × Hb × 1.34) + (0.003 × Pa_{O_2})], and EOR = V_{O_2}/D_{O_2}, then after simplification: EOR = (Sa_{O_2} − Sv_{O_2})/Sa_{O_2}.

Consequently, when Sa_{O_2} = 100%, then EOR = 1 − Sv_{O_2} and Sv_{O_2} = 1 − EOR. Thus, Sv_{O_2} can also be a good surrogate for EOR. Clinically, Sv_{O_2} is one of the most used parameters to assess the balance between tissue O_2 supply and O_2 demand and therefore the hemodynamic status of the patient. Sv_{O_2} and central venous O_2 saturation (Scv_{O_2}) have commonly been used for both GDT protocols in severe sepsis and in the operative room (OR). When Scv_{O_2} is low, it reflects that something is wrong and should lead clinicians to understand the reasons for it and to propose an appropriate optimization strategy.

Normally, Vo_2 is maintained constant, whereas Do_2 varies. If Do_2 declines following a decrease in CO or $CaCo_2$, Vo_2 is maintained by a compensatory increase in the oxygen extraction. If Do_2 continues to decrease, a threshold is reached wherein the OER is maximal and cannot increase further (critical Do_2). Any further reduction in Do_2 will lead to tissue hypoxia, anaerobic metabolism, and lactate production (Vo_2 becomes Do_2-dependent).

The understanding and appreciation of this relationship (**Fig. 3**) during critical illness are capital and have led to the proposition that therapies designed to induce a "supra-physiologic" state could be beneficial for tissue perfusion. Specifically, this idea came from Shoemaker and colleagues,[6] who observed that survivors of critical illness had supranormal levels of Do_2 compared with nonsurvivors. Unfortunately, studies comparing supranormal to conventional resuscitation in critically ill patients have been deleterious: Hayes and colleagues[7] found that achieving supranormal values (cardiac index [CI] >4.5 L/min/m², Do_2 >600 mL/min/m², Vo_2 >170 mL/min/m²) increased mortality compared with normal goal levels. Gattinoni and colleagues[8] similarly targeted critically ill patients by using 3 optimization goals: normal CI (2.5–3.5 L/min/m²), supranormal CI (>4.5), or normal Svo_2 (>70%) and found no benefit in achieving supranormal values for cardiac index. A meta-analysis showed that interventions designed to achieve supraphysiologic goals of cardiac index, Do_2, and Vo_2 did not significantly reduce rates of mortality in all critically ill patients.[9] The current conclusion is that Do_2 must be optimized, not maximized. Using that mindset, different therapeutic targets (using the determinants of Do_2) have been proposed to manage patients. How these different strategies have been implemented in clinical practice and in different departments (ICU and OR) through well-defined GDT algorithms and protocols are discussed in the next sections.

GOAL-DIRECTED FLUID THERAPY IN THE INTENSIVE CARE UNIT

As explained in previous sections, the maintenance of adequate Do_2 to meet the demands of various tissues is essential in critical care medicine. The different determinants of Do_2 can be especially impaired in this patient population and the importance of recognizing and treating them correctly should be stressed. Therefore, careful monitoring and adjustment of these variables are required to achieve the best clinical outcome.

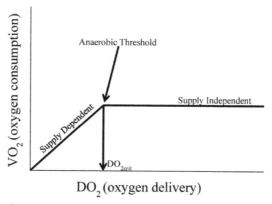

Fig. 3. Relationship between O_2 delivery and consumption: curve showing a defined "knee" where consumption of oxygen by the tissues becomes dependent on delivery.

The first goal in the hemodynamic management of the critically ill patient is to determine the adequacy of tissue/organ perfusion. The evaluation of end-organ delivery of oxygen should first be quickly assessed using broad and widely understood clinical markers (poor peripheral perfusion, altered mental status, and urine output). The details of the other variables are discussed later.

Blood Pressure

Initial hemodynamic management of critically ill patients should include the restoration of blood pressure (BP) with a goal of a mean arterial pressure greater than 65 mm Hg in a previously normotensive patient. This variable must be closely followed because hypotension can lead to impaired cerebral and coronary blood flow (particularly susceptible tissues). A recent trial showed that targeting a mean arterial pressure higher than 65 mm Hg (80–85 mm Hg) in patients with septic shock undergoing resuscitation did not result in significant differences in mortality at either 28 or 90 days.[10] Except for obstructive or cardiogenic shock, volume expansion remains the fundamental treatment to increase intravascular volume. Some clinicians administer an initial fluid bolus (fluid challenge) and assess the effect (increase SV) by measuring static parameters such as central venous pressure (CVP) and/or pulmonary artery occlusion pressure (PAOP). Unfortunately, they think that CVP reflects intravascular volume and that patients with a low CVP are fluid depleted and vice versa. It is well recognized that neither the PAOP nor the CVP can predict ventricular preload and fluid responsiveness.[11]

Volume expansion is important for the initial resuscitation of severe hypotension. Subsequent fluid administration should be given cautiously and only when there is evidence of fluid responsiveness to avoid fluid overload.[12] Indeed, several studies correlate excessive amounts of fluid (positive fluid balance) with increased mortality in acute respiratory distress syndrome or septic patients and failure of weaning from mechanical ventilation.[13–16] Moreover, only 50% of hemodynamically unstable patients are fluid responsive.[17,18]

In contrast to static preload measures, which only rely on hemodynamic values at a given point in time, there are newer dynamic parameters currently available using the change in SV during mechanical ventilation to assess fluid responsiveness. New noninvasive CO monitoring is available today to measure or estimate CO, pulse pressure variation, or SV variation. Resuscitation should, of course, target normalization of BP, HR, and urine output, but also tissue perfusion indices because occult tissue hypoperfusion may persist despite normalization of these vital signs.

BP is not a good indicator of low CO, low Do_2, or hypovolemia: shocked patients may appear adequately resuscitated based on BP even with significant hypoperfusion! That is why other markers of tissue well-being should also be assessed, such as Svo_2, $Scvo_2$, ΔPCo_2, and lactate. They may be also very useful goals of resuscitation when vasopressors are required for persistent hypotension once adequate intravascular volume expansion has been achieved and to evaluate the efficacy of treatment.

Venous Oxygen Saturation

This variable gives an estimation of O_2 saturation of blood returning to the right heart. It is correlated with tissue O_2 extraction and the balance between O_2 delivery and demand. However, it needs a pulmonary artery catheter (PAC), which is very invasive. In this context, $Scvo_2$ may represent an interesting alternative because it can be easily measured by obtaining a blood sample from the central venous catheter. Reinhart and colleagues[19] have shown a good correlation between Svo_2 and $Scvo_2$. Despite this, there is still debate regarding the equivalence between them,[20–23] especially when comparing lower values.[24] However, the surviving Sepsis Campaign recognized the clinical utility of $Scvo_2$ by recommending a Svo_2 of 65% and $Scvo_2$ of 70% in the resuscitation of severe sepsis and septic shock patients.

Arterial Lactate Elevation

This variable is directly proportional to oxygen debt and is commonly taken as an indicator of impaired tissue perfusion because of inadequate O_2 delivery resulting in anaerobic metabolism. It has been shown that during circulatory shock, repeated lactate determinations represent a more reliable prognostic index than an initial value taken alone. Changes in lactate concentration can provide an early and objective evaluation of the patient's response to an intervention.[25] Furthermore, elevation or non-normalization of serum lactate concentration is predictive of adverse outcome in the critically ill patient in shock.[26] Altered levels of serum lactate must also be examined alongside the larger clinical picture because multiple nonhypoxic causes can also result in lactic acidosis, including renal or metabolic disturbances.

Difference Between Venous-Arterial Carbon Dioxide Partial Pressure

The difference between venous-arterial carbon dioxide partial pressure (ΔPCo_2) has also been used to guide the treatment of shock. In the absence of a shunt, Co_2 from the venous blood must be higher than from the arterial blood. The ΔPCo_2 may be a marker of the global hemodynamic status. For example, ΔPCo_2 has been shown to be an indirect marker of the adequacy of systemic flow, which allows for more directed resuscitation.[27] The Fick equation applied to Co_2 indicates that combing $\Delta PCo_2 = CvCo_2 - CaCo_2$ with $VCo_2 = CO \times (CvCo_2 - CaCo_2)$ leads to $\Delta PCo_2 = VCo_2 \times k/CO$ (k is constant) and further indicates that ΔPCo_2 is proportionally related to Co_2 production and inversely proportional to CO.[28] Therefore, with all other variables constant, if CO is low, ΔPCo_2 is high (>6 mm Hg).[29] Vallee and colleagues[30] found that patients with a ΔPCo_2 higher than 6 mm Hg had worse prognosis when compared with those with lower than 6 mm Hg, despite a $Scvo_2$ greater than 70% in both groups. **Fig. 4** gives example of the algorithm used in the critically ill patient to guide therapy based on $Scvo_2$ and ΔPCo_2.

Using the above physiologic variables, a "goal-oriented" protocol of resuscitation seems encouraging. In fact, Rivers and colleagues[31] published a study 13 years ago showing that an early aggressive goal-directed resuscitation protocol (EGDT) administered in the emergency setting reduced mortality from septic shock by 16%. In the ICU and in the emergency department, the Rivers protocol (**Fig. 5**) for the management of the septic patient has been widely accepted. This protocol relies on the early optimization (within 6 hours following the diagnosis of sepsis) of mean arterial pressure, CVP, and $Scvo_2$. The 3 interventions used in this protocol are volume expansion to keep CVP between 8 and 12 mm Hg, vasopressors to maintain mean arterial pressure between 65 and 90 mm Hg, and transfusion and/or inotropes to keep $Scvo_2$ more than 70%.

Over the last decade, multiple investigations have validated the end points used in EGDT.[32] In addition, more than 50 studies and 3 meta-analyses have repeatedly shown the same or better outcome benefits than the original study (18%) in patients of similar illness severity.[33–41] This robust mortality reduction has also been accompanied by a modulation of systemic inflammation,[42] decreases in the progression of organ failure,[43] and decreased health care resource consumption (20% decrease in hospital costs).[44–47] However, a newly published multicenter randomized trial found no significant advantage in morbidity or mortality when comparing a protocol-based resuscitation to standard care in septic shock patients.[48] It puts into question the

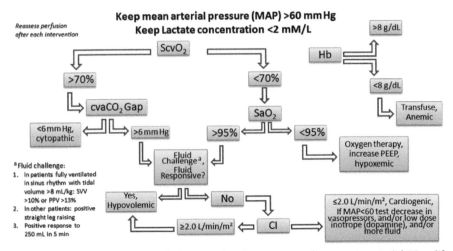

Fig. 4. The Scvo₂-cvaCo₂ gap-guided protocol. cvCo₂gap, central venous-to-arterial PCo₂ difference; PEEP, positive end-expiratory pressure. (*Data from* Vallet B, Pinsky MR, Cecconi M. Resuscitation of patients with septic shock: please "mind the gap"! Intensive Care Med 2013;39(9):1653–5.)

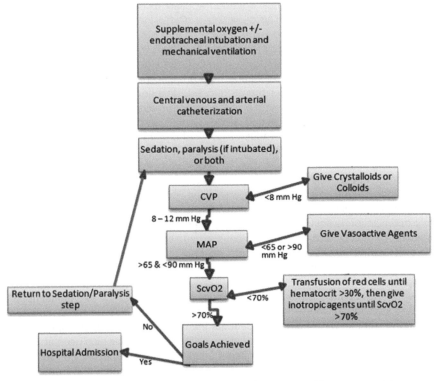

Fig. 5. GDT protocol developed by Emmanuel Rivers for sepsis. MAP, mean arterial pressure. (*Data from* Rivers E, Nguyen B, Havstad S, et al. Early goal-directed therapy in the treatment of severe sepsis and septic shock. N Engl J Med 2001;345(19):1368–77.)

"EGDT approach" in critically ill patients and will surely stimulate more research and exploration into the issue.

Even with a validated resuscitation algorithm, a physiologic approach should still be used to maintain a BP that will sustain vital organ perfusion and optimize blood flow. If possible, this approach should be individualized using noninvasive monitoring to address individual variations. Once again, no monitoring device can replace the close observation of clinical variables and "no monitoring device can improve outcome unless coupled to a treatment which itself improves outcome."[49]

INTRAOPERATIVE GOAL-DIRECTED THERAPY FOR HIGH-RISK SURGICAL PATIENTS

It is estimated that about 240 million anesthesia procedures are performed each year around the world.[50] Among them, 24 million ($\sim$10%) are conducted in "high-risk" patients. Although it can be considered a small percentage of the whole population, one must remember that this sample accounts for more than 80% of the overall mortality related to surgery.[51] Moderate-risk surgery is much more common and represents approximately 40% of the whole population (96 million patients a year). Thankfully, most of these patients present with uncomplicated postoperative course. However, it is estimated that approximately 30% of them ($\sim$29 million patients a year) present with a "minor" postoperative complication, most commonly a gut injury inducing delayed enteral feeding, abdominal distension, nausea, vomiting, or wound complications, such as wound dehiscence or pus from the operation wound.[52] Even if these complications are said to be "minor," they still induce increased postoperative medication, increased length of stay (LOS) in the hospital, and an increase in the cost of the medico-surgical management. In most of these patients, postoperative complications are related to tissue hypoperfusion and inadequate perioperative resuscitation.[52,53]

Upgrading surgical patients from moderate risk to high risk depends on surgical and patient-related factors. High-risk surgical patients are those with an individual mortality risk greater than 5% or undergoing a surgery carrying a mortality of 5%. These patients commonly have a limited cardiopulmonary reserve and an inability to meet the increased oxygen demand imposed by the perioperative surgical stress during major surgery, which is associated with a significant mortality risk.

In addition to these patient-specific risk factors, perioperative risk factors include multiple interventions that can negatively influence the balance between oxygen demand and consumption. Nociceptive surgical stimulations, volume variations due to acute blood losses or transfusions, and administration of anesthetic agent can significantly influence this Vo_2-Do_2 relationship. Some studies evaluated the Vo_2-Do_2 relationship in major surgery[54-56] and showed a decreased capacity for tissue O_2 extraction, which may have led to tissue hypoxia.[57] These observations demonstrate the importance of adequately evaluating the Do_2-Vo_2 relationship in conjunction with the patient's metabolic demand, which is once again strongly affected by surgical conditions.

Initially, significant perioperative cardiopulmonary optimization information came from observational data published by Shoemaker and colleagues[58] 30 years ago. They recognized that, during the perioperative period, the patient developed an "oxygen debt" (imbalance between global Do_2 and Vo_2). If their cardiopulmonary reserve was limited, they were less likely to meet the increased oxygen demand incurred during major surgery.[59] They used predefined hemodynamic measures (Do_2 index) to guide therapy and observed that patients who survived major surgery had higher Do_2 values than nonsurvivors. Using these data, an early GDT aimed at supra-optimizing postoperative Do_2 resulted in lowered complications, LOS, mechanical ventilation, and overall cost. The patients who experienced postoperative complications tended to be those that could also not increase their CO to meet the increased demand of surgery. However, this approach is not beneficial to every high-risk surgical patient because their level of oxygen demand, degree of cardiac function alteration, and capacities of oxygen extraction may significantly vary. Thus, the major concern of the anesthetist in the perioperative period is to optimize the patient's *individual* volemic status by aiming to achieve well-defined goals (based on flow-related parameters such as SV) to maximize end-organ Do_2.

Several studies have demonstrated that CO optimization during high-risk surgery has the ability to improve postoperative patient outcome while also decreasing the cost of surgery.[60–63] However, recent survey studies suggest that goal-directed fluid management is poorly adopted in clinical practice.[3] Most anesthetists use the combination of formulas and fixed-volume calculations with vital sign optimization (BP, HR, CVP, urine output) to guide their perioperative fluid therapy. Le Manach and colleagues[64] showed that changes in BP cannot be used to track changes in SV induced by volume expansion. Consequently, optimization of Do_2 to the tissues during surgery cannot be conducted by monitoring arterial pressure alone. Because arterial pressure and CO both depend on systemic vascular resistance, a normal or even supranormal arterial pressure does not guarantee an adequate CO.

Ideally, one would like to monitor the volume change instead of the pressure change. However, although flow measuring technology is steadily improving, it is still not as technologically straightforward as pressure measurements. Outside of such CO monitoring devices, new parameters (called functional hemodynamic parameters) have been developed and used much more commonly. These parameters can be obtained from arterial pressure waveforms (pulse pressure variation or SV variation) and rely on cardiopulmonary interactions in patients undergoing general anesthesia on mechanical ventilation.[65,66]

As is known, hypovolemia induces hypotension, oliguria, and tachycardia. That is a fact. However, one has to be very careful: these signs are not related to all levels of hypovolemia. They are related to severe hypovolemia![67,68] Moreover, they are not specific and can be present even in the absence of hypovolemia. They are therefore neither sensitive nor specific and should not be used independently for assessing a patient's fluid status. In addition, CVP and pulmonary capillary wedge pressure (PCWP) have been used for years for monitoring a patient's volume status. Unfortunately, almost all the studies focusing on the ability of CVP and PCWP to predict fluid responsiveness have failed to demonstrate any accuracy of these parameters for predicting the effects of volume expansion on CO.[69]

In fact, the main question the anesthesiologist has to answer before performing volume expansion is, "will my patient increase cardiac output in response?" or, more correctly, "is my patient preload dependent?". Preload dependence is defined as the ability of the heart to increase SV in response to an increase in preload. To understand this concept, the Frank-Starling relationship has to be revisited. This relationship links preload to SV and presents 2 distinct parts: a steep portion and a plateau. If the patient is on the steep portion of the Frank-Starling relationship, then an increase in preload (induced by volume expansion) is going to induce an important increase in SV. Alternatively, if the patient is on the plateau of this relationship, then increasing preload will have no effect on SV. Moreover, the Frank-Starling relationship does not only depend on preload and SV but also depends on cardiac function. When cardiac function is impaired, the Frank-Starling relationship is flattened and for the same level of preload the effects of volume expansion on SV are going to be less significant. This concept further explains why preload parameters such as CVP or PCWP are not accurate predictors of fluid responsiveness.

Instead of monitoring a given parameter, functional hemodynamic monitoring assesses the effects of a stressor on commonly recorded variables.[49] For the assessment of preload dependence, the stress is a "fluid challenge" and the parameter is SV. In mechanically ventilated patients under general anesthesia, the effects of positive pressure ventilation on preload and SV are used to detect fluid responsiveness. If mechanical ventilation induces important respiratory variations in stroke volume (SVV) or in arterial pulse pressure (PPV), it is more likely that the patient is preload-dependent.[5] These dynamic parameters (SVV, PPV) have consistently been shown to be superior to static parameters (CVP, PCWP) for the prediction of fluid responsiveness. Our best clinical evidence currently demonstrates that CVP and PCWP, as well as oliguria, hypotension, and tachycardia, should not be used for predicting the effects of volume expansion on CO.[17,69]

Dynamic parameters of fluid responsiveness based on cardiopulmonary interactions have several limitations that need to be clearly stated before they can be adequately used in the clinical setting. First, these parameters have to be used in mechanically ventilated patients under general anesthesia. Up to now, studies conducted in spontaneously breathing patients failed to demonstrate that PPV can predict fluid responsiveness.[70] Moreover, tidal volume has an impact on the predictive value of PPV and a tidal volume of 8 mL/kg of body weight is required.[71] In addition, patients have to be in sinus rhythm; chest must be closed (open chest as well as open pericardium strongly modify the cardiopulmonary interactions), and intra-abdominal pressure has to be within normal ranges.[72] Unfortunately, only 39% of the patients undergoing surgical procedures in the OR met the criteria for the monitoring of fluid responsiveness using noninvasively measured PPV.[73] Also, despite a strong predictive value, PPV may be in the inconclusive "gray zone" (between 9% and 13%) in approximately 25% of patients during general anesthesia.[74]

The use of flow-related parameters to guide intraoperative goal-directed fluid therapy has appeal because these parameters provide a numeric representation of the patient's volume status, which can be difficult to ascertain using standard monitors, urine output, or even CVP.[69,75,76] **Fig. 6** demonstrates an example of a GDT algorithm using SVV and PPV in the OR. Gan and colleagues[60] in 2002 reported earlier return to bowel function, lower incidence of postoperative nausea and vomiting, and decrease in length of postoperative hospital stay with the use of the esophageal Doppler to maximize SV. Intraoperative GDT has also been reported to improve outcome following surgery in high-risk patients by decreasing both morbidity and hospital LOS.[77–80] Previously published studies have shown decreased complications and hospital LOS in high-risk patients undergoing major abdominal surgery with SVV-guided GDT therapy.[63,81] In addition, similar results have been shown in non-high-risk surgical patients undergoing elective total hip arthroplasty[82] and major abdominal surgery.[83] **Table 2** lists the major studies demonstrating that goal-directed therapy is associated with decreased postoperative complications associated with GDT when compared with more conventional fluid management.

In addition, Svo_2 can provide information about Vo_2 and can be used to calculate CO through a pulmonary catheter. A study of cardiac surgery patients found that GDT aimed at normalizing Svo_2 (>70%) and lactate (<2 mmol/L) in the first 8 hours after surgery demonstrated decreased LOS and perioperative organ dysfunction.[84] Unfortunately, Svo_2 has the disadvantage of requiring a PAC, which comes with its own inherent risks.[85] $Scvo_2$, taken from a catheter in the internal jugular or subclavian vein, has also been shown to parallel Svo_2.[19,86] Donati and colleagues[87] demonstrated improved outcome in patients treated with GDT using fluids and dobutamine titrated to optimize oxygen extraction (ERo_2) at less than 27% ($Scvo_2$ >73%). Reductions in $Scvo_2$ in the perioperative setting are independently associated with a higher risk of

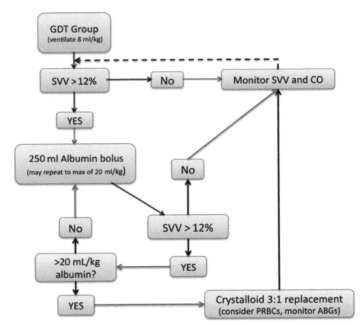

Fig. 6. GDT protocol based on PPV/SVV alone. ABG, arterial blood gas; PRBC, packed red blood cells. (*Adapted from* Ramsingh DS, Sanghvi C, Gamboa J, et al. Outcome impact of goal directed fluid therapy during high risk abdominal surgery in low to moderate risk patients: a randomized controlled trial. J Clin Monit Comput 2013;27(3):51; with permission.)

postoperative complications.[88] The central venous to arterial carbon dioxide difference $P(v - a)Co_2$ has been proposed by some authors for assessment of tissue perfusion.[30,89] Values of $P(v - a)Co_2$ larger than 6 mm Hg were found to be associated with poor outcome and organ dysfunctions.[27,30] Other markers, such as as lactate serum,[90,91] base deficit, and tissue hypercarbia, require further investigation as GDT end points before conclusions can be drawn in high-risk surgery.

Finally, high-risk surgical patients have been shown to benefit from CO optimization using semi-invasive technologies. Unfortunately, a recent survey with the American Society of Anesthesiology and the European Society of Anesthesiology showed a considerable gap between accumulating evidence about the benefits of perioperative hemodynamic optimization and the available technologies that may facilitate its clinical implementation and clinical practices in both Europe and the United States.[3] In the future, GDT using more sophisticated and less invasive monitoring will help clinicians optimize their patients' hemodynamic status during surgery. In Irvine (California), a novel-closed loop fluid administration system and hemodynamic management system based on SV monitoring and optimization (Learning Intravenous Resuscitator) has recently been described.[92,93] The aim of this system is to ease implementation of protocols in clinical settings and to apply goal-directed fluid therapy protocols automatically. After conducting simulation,[92,93] engineering,[94] and animal studies,[95] it is now starting to be used in the OR.[96] The system is designed to titrate fluid administration until SV reaches the plateau of the Frank-Starling relationship and then maintain that plateau throughout patient care. To achieve this goal, the closed loop system monitors SV, tracks volume expansion–induced changes in SV, and uses pulse pressure variation or SV variation to refine fluid responsiveness predictions.[64,74] Future studies will help to evaluate the real benefits of this system.

Table 2
Comparison of perioperative goal-directed therapy research studies during major surgeries

Author	Surgical Type	Patient	Timing	Guiding Goals	Results
Benes et al,[102] 2010	Major abdominal	120	Intraoperative	SVV	↓ Complications and hospital LOS
Goepfert et al,[103] 2013	Cardiac	100	Postoperative	SVV	↓ Complications and ICU LOS
Mayer et al,[63] 2010	Major abdominal	60	Intraoperative	SVV	↓ Complications and hospital LOS No difference in ICU LOS
Ramsingh et al,[104] 2013	Major abdominal	38	Intraoperative	SVV	Faster return of GI function and ↓ hospital LOS
Scheeren et al,[105] 2013	Major abdominal	64	Intraoperative	SVV	↓ Infections in surgical sites
Zheng et al,[106] 2013	Major abdominal	60	Intraoperative	SVV	Faster return of GI function and ↓ hospital LOS and ICU LOS
Lopes et al,[107] 2007	Major abdominal	33	Intraoperative	PPV	↓ Complications and hospital LOS and ICU LOS, ↓ time of mechanical ventilation
Salzwedel et al,[108] 2013	Major abdominal	160	Intraoperative	PPV	↓ Complications, no difference in ICU LOS
Zhang et al,[109] 2012	Major abdominal	60	Intraoperative	PPV	Faster return of GI function and ↓ hospital LOS
Mythen & Webb,[110] 1995	Cardiac surgery	60	Intraoperative	ED/CVP	↑ Gut mucosal perfusion ↓ Complications, hospital LOS, and ICU LOS
Wackeling et al,[62] 2005	Major abdominal	128	Intraoperative	ED/CVP	↑ Gut function recovery ↓ GI complications and hospital LOS
Conway et al,[111] 2002	Major abdominal	55	Intraoperative	ED	↓* Complications, ↓ ICU LOS admissions, ↑* hospital LOS
McKendry et al,[112] 2004	Cardiac	174	Postoperative	ED	↓ Hospital LOS, ↓* ICU LOS, ↓* major complications and death
Buettner et al,[113] 2008	Major abdominal and gynecologic	80	Intraoperative	PICCO	No difference in ICU LOS, hospital LOS, morbi-mortality
Pearse et al,[61] 2005	Major general surgery	122	Postoperative	LidCO + Do₂	↓ Complications and hospital LOS
Donati et al,[87] 2007	Major abdominal	135	Intraoperative	ERo₂ < 27%	↓ Postoperative organ failure and hospital LOS No difference in mortality
Polonen et al,[84] 2000	Cardiac surgery	393	Postoperative	Svo₂ > 70%	↓ Morbidity

Abbreviations: ↓, decrease with P<.05; ↑, increase with P<.05; ↓*, decrease with P>.05; ↑*, increase with P>.05; ED, esophageal Doppler; PICCO, pulse induced contour cardiac output.

SUMMARY

When evaluating the critically ill patient in need of fluid management, GDT has mounted strong clinical evidence to support its extensive use. Despite these favorable results, widespread implementation of GDT has not yet been accomplished. Recently, significant progress has been made; most notably, recommendations have been published in the United Kingdom (Enhanced Recovery Partnership), France (French Society of Anesthesiology), and Europe (Enhanced Recovery After Surgery Society).[97,98] Some of the most significant progress has been made in the United Kingdom, where the National Health Service has created financial incentives to ensure hospitals implement hemodynamic optimization in at least 80% of eligible patients. Further creation and implementation of institutional GDT standards are necessary to minimize variability.

As seen by the multiple paths of research discussed above, there is still no universal consensus on an optimal end point for GDT in critically ill patients. As in other areas of medicine, when this occurs, providers must move toward a more "individualized approach" to ensure proper patient care. Hemodynamic optimization in the ICU and OR needs more than BP, HR, CVP, and urine output monitoring. It is essential to monitor dynamic parameters of fluid responsiveness (SV, PPV, and SVV) and CO as minimally invasively as possible. All of these small improvements and standardizations will provide a better hemodynamic assessment of patient status and ultimately improve outcome.

REFERENCES

1. Guyton AH, Hall JE. Heart muscle; the heart as a pump and function of the heart valves. In: Textbook of medical physiology. 11th edition. Philadelphia: Elsevier, Inc; Saunders Elsevier; 2006. p. 103–15.
2. Guyton AH, Hall JE. Overview of the circulation: medical physics of pressure, flow, and resistance. In: Textbook of medical physiology. 11th edition. Philadelphia: Elsevier, Inc; Saunders Elsevier; 2006. p. 161–70.
3. Cannesson M, Pestel G, Ricks C, et al. Hemodynamic monitoring and management in patients undergoing high risk surgery: a survey among North American and European anesthesiologists. Crit Care 2011;15(4):R197.
4. Miller TE, Roche AM, Gan TJ. Poor adoption of hemodynamic optimization during major surgery: are we practicing substandard care? Anesth Analg 2011;112(6):1274–6.
5. Cannesson M. Arterial pressure variation and goal-directed fluid therapy. J Cardiothorac Vasc Anesth 2010;24(3):487–97.
6. Shoemaker WC, Appel PL, Kram HB, et al. Prospective trial of supranormal values of survivors as therapeutic goals in high-risk surgical patients. Chest 1988;94(6):1176–86.
7. Hayes MA, Timmins AC, Yau EH, et al. Elevation of systemic oxygen delivery in the treatment of critically ill patients. N Engl J Med 1994;330(24):1717–22.
8. Gattinoni L, Brazzi L, Pelosi P, et al. A trial of goal-oriented hemodynamic therapy in critically ill patients. SvO2 Collaborative Group. N Engl J Med 1995; 333(16):1025–32.
9. Heyland DK, Cook DJ, King D, et al. Maximizing oxygen delivery in critically ill patients: a methodologic appraisal of the evidence. Crit Care Med 1996;24(3): 517–24.
10. Asfar P, Meziani F, Hamel JF, et al. High versus low blood-pressure target in patients with septic shock. N Engl J Med 2014;370(17):1583–93.

11. Osman D, Ridel C, Ray P, et al. Cardiac filling pressures are not appropriate to predict hemodynamic response to volume challenge. Crit Care Med 2007;35(1):64–8.
12. Vincent JL, Weil MH. Fluid challenge revisited. Crit Care Med 2006;34(5):1333–7.
13. Humphrey H, Hall J, Sznajder I, et al. Improved survival in ARDS patients associated with a reduction in pulmonary capillary wedge pressure. Chest 1990;97(5):1176–80.
14. Simmons RS, Berdine GG, Seidenfeld JJ, et al. Fluid balance and the adult respiratory distress syndrome. Am Rev Respir Dis 1987;135(4):924–9.
15. Alsous F, Khamiees M, DeGirolamo A, et al. Negative fluid balance predicts survival in patients with septic shock: a retrospective pilot study. Chest 2000;117(6):1749–54.
16. Upadya A, Tilluckdharry L, Muralidharan V, et al. Fluid balance and weaning outcomes. Intensive Care Med 2005;31(12):1643–7.
17. Marik PE, Cavallazzi R, Vasu T, et al. Dynamic changes in arterial waveform derived variables and fluid responsiveness in mechanically ventilated patients: a systematic review of the literature. Crit Care Med 2009;37(9):2642–7.
18. Michard F, Teboul JL. Predicting fluid responsiveness in ICU patients: a critical analysis of the evidence. Chest 2002;121(6):2000–8.
19. Reinhart K, Kuhn HJ, Hartog C, et al. Continuous central venous and pulmonary artery oxygen saturation monitoring in the critically ill. Intensive Care Med 2004;30(8):1572–8.
20. Ladakis C, Myrianthefs P, Karabinis A, et al. Central venous and mixed venous oxygen saturation in critically ill patients. Respiration 2001;68(3):279–85.
21. Chawla LS, Zia H, Gutierrez G, et al. Lack of equivalence between central and mixed venous oxygen saturation. Chest 2004;126(6):1891–6.
22. Edwards JD, Mayall RM. Importance of the sampling site for measurement of mixed venous oxygen saturation in shock. Crit Care Med 1998;26(8):1356–60.
23. Reinhart K, Zia H, Gutierrez G, et al. Comparison of central-venous to mixed-venous oxygen saturation during changes in oxygen supply/demand. Chest 1989;95(6):1216–21.
24. Rivers E. Mixed vs central venous oxygen saturation may be not numerically equal, but both are still clinically useful. Chest 2006;129(3):507–8.
25. Vincent JL, Dufaye P, Berre J, et al. Serial lactate determinations during circulatory shock. Crit Care Med 1983;11(6):449–51.
26. Suistomaa M, Ruokonen E, Kari A, et al. Time-pattern of lactate and lactate to pyruvate ratio in the first 24 hours of intensive care emergency admissions. Shock 2000;14(1):8–12.
27. Bakker J, Vincent JL, Gris P, et al. Veno-arterial carbon dioxide gradient in human septic shock. Chest 1992;101(2):509–15.
28. Monnet X, Julien F, Ait-Hamou N, et al. Lactate and venoarterial carbon dioxide difference/arterial-venous oxygen difference ratio, but not central venous oxygen saturation, predict increase in oxygen consumption in fluid responders. Crit Care Med 2013;41(6):1412–20.
29. Lamia B, Monnet X, Teboul JL. Meaning of arterio-venous PCO2 difference in circulatory shock. Minerva Anestesiol 2006;72(6):597–604.
30. Vallee F, Vallet B, Mathe O, et al. Central venous-to-arterial carbon dioxide difference: an additional target for goal-directed therapy in septic shock? Intensive Care Med 2008;34(12):2218–25.
31. Rivers E, Nguyen B, Havstad S, et al. Early goal-directed therapy in the treatment of severe sepsis and septic shock. N Engl J Med 2001;345(19):1368–77.

32. Varpula M, Tallgren M, Saukkonen K, et al. Hemodynamic variables related to outcome in septic shock. Intensive Care Med 2005;31:1066–71.

33. Rivers EP, Katranji M, Jaehne KA, et al. Early interventions in severe sepsis and septic shock: a review of the evidence one decade later. Minerva Anestesiol 2012;78(6):712–24.

34. Rivers EP, Coba V, Whitmill M. Early goal-directed therapy in severe sepsis and septic shock: a contemporary review of the literature. Curr Opin Anaesthesiol 2008;21(2):128–40.

35. Jones AE, Brown MD, Trzeciak S, et al. The effect of a quantitative resuscitation strategy on mortality in patients with sepsis: a meta-analysis. Crit Care Med 2008;36(10):2734–9.

36. Dellinger RP, Levy MM, Carlet JM, et al. Surviving Sepsis Campaign: international guidelines for management of severe sepsis and septic shock: 2008. Crit Care Med 2008;36(1):296–327.

37. Townsend SR, Schorr C, Levy MM, et al. Reducing mortality in severe sepsis: the surviving sepsis campaign. Clin Chest Med 2008;29(4):721–33.

38. Rivers EP, Coba V, Rudis M. Standardized order sets for the treatment of severe sepsis and septic shock. Expert Rev Anti Infect Ther 2009;7(9):1075–9.

39. Chamberlain DJ, Willis EM, Bersten AB. The severe sepsis bundles as processes of care: a meta-analysis. Aust Crit Care 2011;24(4):229–43.

40. Reinhart K, Bloos F. The value of venous oximetry. Curr Opin Crit Care 2005;11(3):259–63.

41. Wang AT, Liu F, Zhu X, et al. The effect of an optimized resuscitation strategy on prognosis of patients with septic shock: a systematic review. Zhongguo Wei Zhong Bing Ji Jiu Yi Xue 2012;24(1):13–7 [in Chinese].

42. Rivers EP, Kruse JA, Jacobsen G, et al. The influence of early hemodynamic optimization on biomarker patterns of severe sepsis and septic shock. Crit Care Med 2007;35(9):2016–24.

43. Kiers HD, Kruse JA, Jacobsen G, et al. Effect of early achievement of physiologic resuscitation goals in septic patients admitted from the ward on the kidneys. J Crit Care 2010;25(4):563–9.

44. Shorr AF, Kruse JA, Jacobsen G, et al. Economic implications of an evidence-based sepsis protocol: can we improve outcomes and lower costs? Crit Care Med 2007;35(5):1257–62.

45. Talmor D, Kruse JA, Jacobsen G, et al. The costs and cost-effectiveness of an integrated sepsis treatment protocol. Crit Care Med 2008;36(4):1168–74.

46. Jones AE, Troyer JL, Kline JA. Cost-effectiveness of an emergency department-based early sepsis resuscitation protocol. Crit Care Med 2011;39(6):1306–12.

47. Suarez D, Ferrer R, Artigas A, et al. Cost-effectiveness of the Surviving Sepsis Campaign protocol for severe sepsis: a prospective nation-wide study in Spain. Intensive Care Med 2011;37(3):444–52.

48. A randomized trial of protocol-based care for early septic shock. N Engl J Med 2014;370(18):1683–93.

49. Pinsky MR, Payen D. Functional hemodynamic monitoring. Crit Care 2005;9(6):566–72.

50. Weiser TG, Regenbogen SE, Thompson KD, et al. An estimation of the global volume of surgery: a modelling strategy based on available data. Lancet 2008;372(9633):139–44.

51. Pearse RM, Harrison DA, James P, et al. Identification and characterisation of the high-risk surgical population in the United Kingdom. Crit Care 2006;10(3):R81.

52. Bennett-Guerrero E, Welsby I, Dunn TJ, et al. The use of a postoperative morbidity survey to evaluate patients with prolonged hospitalization after routine, moderate-risk, elective surgery. Anesth Analg 1999;89:514–9.
53. Gan TJ, Mythen MG. Does peroperative gut-mucosa hypoperfusion cause post-operative nausea and vomiting? Lancet 1995;345(8957):1123–4.
54. Lugo G, Arizpe D, Dominguez G, et al. Relationship between oxygen consumption and oxygen delivery during anesthesia in high-risk surgical patients. Crit Care Med 1993;21(1):64–9.
55. Shibutani K, Komatsu T, Kubal K, et al. Critical level of oxygen delivery in anesthetized man. Crit Care Med 1983;11(8):640–3.
56. Waxman K, Nolan LS, Shoemaker WC. Sequential perioperative lactate determination. Physiological and clinical implications. Crit Care Med 1982;10(2):96–9.
57. Shoemaker WC, Appel PL, Kram HB. Tissue oxygen debt as a determinant of lethal and nonlethal postoperative organ failure. Crit Care Med 1988;16(11):1117–20.
58. Shoemaker WC, Appel P, Bland R. Use of physiologic monitoring to predict outcome and to assist in clinical decisions in critically ill postoperative patients. Am J Surg 1983;146(1):43–50.
59. Shoemaker WC, Appel PL, Kram HB. Role of oxygen debt in the development of organ failure sepsis, and death in high-risk surgical patients. Chest 1992;102(1):208–15.
60. Gan TJ, Soppitt A, Maroof M, et al. Goal-directed intraoperative fluid administration reduces length of hospital stay after major surgery. Anesthesiology 2002;97(4):820–6.
61. Pearse R, Dawson D, Fawcett J, et al. Early goal-directed therapy after major surgery reduces complications and duration of hospital stay. A randomised, controlled trial [ISRCTN38797445]. Crit Care 2005;9(6):R687–93.
62. Wakeling HG, McFall MR, Jenkins CS, et al. Intraoperative oesophageal Doppler guided fluid management shortens postoperative hospital stay after major bowel surgery. Br J Anaesth 2005;95(5):634–42.
63. Mayer J, Boldt J, Mengistu AM, et al. Goal-directed intraoperative therapy based on autocalibrated arterial pressure waveform analysis reduces hospital stay in high-risk surgical patients: a randomized, controlled trial. Crit Care 2010;14(1):R18.
64. Le Manach Y, Hofer CK, Lehot JJ, et al. Can changes in arterial pressure be used to detect changes in cardiac output during volume expansion in the perioperative period? Anesthesiology 2012;117(6):1165–74.
65. Cannesson M, Slieker J, Desebbe O, et al. The ability of a novel algorithm for automatic estimation of the respiratory variations in arterial pulse pressure to monitor fluid responsiveness in the operating room. Anesth Analg 2008;106(4):1195–200 [table of contents].
66. Michard F, Boussat S, Chemla D, et al. Relation between respiratory changes in arterial pulse pressure and fluid responsiveness in septic patients with acute circulatory failure. Am J Respir Crit Care Med 2000;162(1):134–8.
67. Perel A, Pizov R, Cotev S. Systolic blood pressure variation is a sensitive indicator of hypovolemia in ventilated dogs subjected to graded hemorrhage. Anesthesiology 1987;67(4):498–502.
68. Vatner SF, Braunwald E. Cardiovascular control mechanisms in the conscious state. N Engl J Med 1975;293(19):970–6.
69. Marik PE, Baram M, Vahid B. Does central venous pressure predict fluid responsiveness?: a systematic review of the literature and the tale of seven mares. Chest 2008;134(1):172–8.

70. De Backer D, Pinsky MR. Can one predict fluid responsiveness in spontaneously breathing patients? Intensive Care Med 2007;33(7):1111–3.

71. De Backer D, Heenen S, Piagnerelli M, et al. Pulse pressure variations to predict fluid responsiveness: influence of tidal volume. Intensive Care Med 2005;31(4): 517–23.

72. Duperret S, Lhuillier F, Piriou V, et al. Increased intra-abdominal pressure affects respiratory variations in arterial pressure in normovolaemic and hypovolaemic mechanically ventilated pigs. Intensive Care Med 2007;33:163–71.

73. Maguire S, Rinehart J, Vakharia S, et al. Technical communication: respiratory variation in pulse pressure and plethysmographic waveforms: intraoperative applicability in a North American academic center. Anesth Analg 2011;112(1): 94–6.

74. Cannesson M, Le Manach Y, Hofer CK, et al. Assessing the diagnostic accuracy of pulse pressure variations for the prediction of fluid responsiveness: a "gray zone" approach. Anesthesiology 2011;115(2):231–41.

75. Gelman S. Venous function and central venous pressure: a physiologic story. Anesthesiology 2008;108(4):735–48.

76. Howell MD, Donnino M, Clardy P, et al. Occult hypoperfusion and mortality in patients with suspected infection. Intensive Care Med 2007;33(11):1892–9.

77. Abbas SM, Hill AG. Systematic review of the literature for the use of oesophageal Doppler monitor for fluid replacement in major abdominal surgery. Anaesthesia 2008;63(1):44–51.

78. Bundgaard-Nielsen M, Holte K, Secher NH, et al. Monitoring of peri-operative fluid administration by individualized goal-directed therapy. Acta Anaesthesiol Scand 2007;51(3):331–40.

79. Giglio MT, Marucci M, Testini M, et al. Goal-directed haemodynamic therapy and gastrointestinal complications in major surgery: a meta-analysis of randomized controlled trials. Br J Anaesth 2009;103(5):637–46.

80. Rahbari NN, Marucci M, Testini M, et al. Meta-analysis of standard, restrictive and supplemental fluid administration in colorectal surgery. Br J Surg 2009; 96(4):331–41.

81. Lees N, Hamilton M, Rhodes A. Clinical review: goal-directed therapy in high risk surgical patients. Crit Care 2009;13(5):231.

82. Cecconi M, Fasano N, Langiano N, et al. Goal-directed haemodynamic therapy during elective total hip arthroplasty under regional anaesthesia. Crit Care 2011; 15(3):R132.

83. Ramsingh D, Applegate II. Evaluation of the Use of Arterial Pulse Waveform Contour Analysis (PWCA) for Goal Directed Therapy in Low/Moderate Risk Patients Undergoing Major Abdominal Surgery. American Society of Anesthesiologists Meeting 2010. 2010.

84. Polonen P, Ruokonen E, Hippelainen M, et al. A prospective, randomized study of goal-oriented hemodynamic therapy in cardiac surgical patients. Anesth Analg 2000;90(5):1052–9.

85. Bowdle TA. Complications of invasive monitoring. Anesthesiol Clin North America 2002;20(3):571–88.

86. Dueck MH, Klimek M, Appenrodt S, et al. Trends but not individual values of central venous oxygen saturation agree with mixed venous oxygen saturation during varying hemodynamic conditions. Anesthesiology 2005;103(2):249–57.

87. Donati A, Loggi S, Preiser JC, et al. Goal-directed intraoperative therapy reduces morbidity and length of hospital stay in high-risk surgical patients. Chest 2007;132(6):1817–24.

88. Pearse R, Dawson D, Fawcett J, et al. Changes in central venous saturation after major surgery, and association with outcome. Crit Care 2005;9(6):R694–9.

89. Futier E, Robin E, Jabaudon M, et al. Central venous O(2) saturation and venous-to-arterial CO(2) difference as complementary tools for goal-directed therapy during high-risk surgery. Crit Care 2010;14(5):R193.

90. Jones AE, Shapiro NI, Trzeciak S, et al. Lactate clearance vs central venous oxygen saturation as goals of early sepsis therapy: a randomized clinical trial. JAMA 2010;303(8):739–46.

91. Wenkui Y, Ning L, Jianfeng G, et al. Restricted peri-operative fluid administration adjusted by serum lactate level improved outcome after major elective surgery for gastrointestinal malignancy. Surgery 2010;147(4):542–52.

92. Rinehart J, Alexander B, Le Manach Y, et al. Evaluation of a novel closed-loop fluid-administration system based on dynamic predictors of fluid responsiveness: an in silico simulation study. Crit Care 2011;15(6):R278.

93. Rinehart J, Chung E, Canales C, et al. Intraoperative stroke volume optimization using stroke volume, arterial pressure, and heart rate: closed-loop (learning intravenous resuscitator) versus anesthesiologists. J Cardiothorac Vasc Anesth 2012;26(5):933–9.

94. Rinehart J, Chung E, Canales C, et al. Closed-loop fluid resuscitation: robustness against weight and cardiac contractility variations. Anesth Analg 2013; 117(5):1110–8.

95. Rinehart J, Lee C, Canales C, et al. Closed-loop fluid administration compared to anesthesiologist management for hemodynamic optimization and resuscitation during surgery: an in vivo study. Anesth Analg 2013; 117(5):1119–29.

96. Rinehart J, Le Manach Y, Douiri H, et al. First closed-loop goal directed fluid therapy during surgery: a pilot study. Ann Fr Anesth Reanim 2014;33(3): e35–41.

97. Vallet B, Blanloeil Y, Cholley B, et al. Guidelines for perioperative haemodynamic optimization. Ann Fr Anesth Reanim 2013;32(10):e151–8.

98. Gustafsson UO, Scott MJ, Schwenk W, et al. Guidelines for perioperative care in elective colonic surgery: Enhanced Recovery After Surgery (ERAS((R))) Society recommendations. World J Surg 2013;37(2):259–84.

99. Murakawa K, Kobayashi A. Effects of vasopressors on renal tissue gas tensions during hemorrhagic shock in dogs. Crit Care Med 1988;16(8):789–92.

100. Rosenberg AL, Dechert RE, Park PK, et al. Review of a large clinical series: association of cumulative fluid balance on outcome in acute lung injury: a retrospective review of the ARDSnet tidal volume study cohort. J Intensive Care Med 2009;24(1):35–46.

101. Chappell D, Jacob M, Hofmann-Kiefer K, et al. A rational approach to perioperative fluid management. Anesthesiology 2008;109(4):723–40.

102. Benes J, Chytra I, Altmann P, et al. Intraoperative fluid optimization using stroke volume variation in high risk surgical patients: results of prospective randomized study. Crit Care 2010;14(3):R118.

103. Goepfert MS, Richter HP, Zu Eulenburg C, et al. Individually optimized hemodynamic therapy reduces complications and length of stay in the intensive care unit: a prospective, randomized controlled trial. Anesthesiology 2013;119(4): 824–36.

104. Ramsingh DS, Sanghvi C, Gamboa J, et al. Outcome impact of goal directed fluid therapy during high risk abdominal surgery in low to moderate risk patients: a randomized controlled trial. J Clin Monit Comput 2013;27(3):249–57.

105. Scheeren TW, Wiesenack C, Gerlach H, et al. Goal-directed intraoperative fluid therapy guided by stroke volume and its variation in high-risk surgical patients: a prospective randomized multicentre study. J Clin Monit Comput 2013;27(3): 225–33.

106. Zheng H, Guo H, Ye JR, et al. Goal-directed fluid therapy in gastrointestinal surgery in older coronary heart disease patients: randomized trial. World J Surg 2013;37(12):2820–9.

107. Lopes MR, Oliveira MA, Pereira VO, et al. Goal-directed fluid management based on pulse pressure variation monitoring during high-risk surgery: a pilot randomized controlled trial. Crit Care 2007;11(5):R100.

108. Salzwedel C, Puig J, Carstens A, et al. Perioperative goal-directed hemodynamic therapy based on radial arterial pulse pressure variation and continuous cardiac index trending reduces postoperative complications after major abdominal surgery: a multi-center, prospective, randomized study. Crit Care 2013; 17(5):R191.

109. Zhang J, Qiao H, He Z, et al. Intraoperative fluid management in open gastrointestinal surgery: goal-directed versus restrictive. Clinics (Sao Paulo) 2012; 67(10):1149–55.

110. Mythen MG, Webb AR. Perioperative plasma volume expansion reduces the incidence of gut mucosal hypoperfusion during cardiac surgery. Arch Surg 1995;130(4):423–9.

111. Conway DH, Mayall R, Abdul-Latif MS, et al. Randomised controlled trial investigating the influence of intravenous fluid titration using oesophageal Doppler monitoring during bowel surgery. Anaesthesia 2002;57(9):845–9.

112. McKendry M, McGloin H, Saberi D, et al. Randomised controlled trial assessing the impact of a nurse delivered, flow monitored protocol for optimisation of circulatory status after cardiac surgery. BMJ 2004;329(7460):258.

113. Buettner M, Schummer W, Huettemann E, et al. Influence of systolic-pressure-variation-guided intraoperative fluid management on organ function and oxygen transport. Br J Anaesth 2008;101(2):194–9.

Using What You Get
Dynamic Physiologic Signatures of Critical Illness

Andre L. Holder, MD, MSc, Gilles Clermont, MD, CM, MSc*

KEYWORDS

- Data hierarchy • Fused parameter • Physiologic signature
- Cardiopulmonary instability • Machine learning

KEY POINTS

- Physiologic monitoring of dynamic changes is more useful than static variables for the early detection of critical illness, and the guidance and appropriate cessation of therapeutic interventions.
- Physiologic monitoring techniques that take advantage of complex organ-organ interaction (eg, heart rate variability, arterial pressure variation, and secondary variables from hemodynamic waveforms) are valuable but are an underused resource for identifying critical illness.
- Using new tools to analyze available physiologic variables, it is possible to construct the physiologic signatures at every point in a disease process to identify and treat critical illness as early as possible.
- Tools that integrate large amounts of physiologic data are complex to develop; their use requires collaboration with information technology experts.
- The integration of physiologic predictors and applications in critical illness is an area of research still under intense investigation.

INTRODUCTION

Cardiopulmonary instability can occur in any disease process when the metabolic needs of the body are not being met with adequate supply. Cardiopulmonary equilibrium is achieved in the presence of adequate oxygenation, preload, contractility, and vasomotor tone. Although the body may be able to compensate for a significant change in any one of these components from baseline, any change may still lead to

The work was supported by: National Institutes of Health grants NR013912, HL07820 and HL67181.
Conflicts of interest: none declared.
Department of Critical Care Medicine, University of Pittsburgh, Pittsburgh, PA, USA
* Corresponding author. 602A Scaife Hall, 3550 Terrace Street, Pittsburgh, PA 15261.
E-mail address: clermontg@ccm.upmc.edu

significant morbidity and mortality. Each component can contribute to cardiopulmonary instability. In the setting of trauma, there is a loss of adequate preload because of hemorrhage. Hemorrhage accounts for 50% of deaths within the first 24 hours of hospitalization for a traumatic injury.[1] Vasomotor tone is the most prominent derangement in sepsis, although these patients can also experience hypovolemia with reduced preload and decreased contractility because of myocardial suppression. Inflammatory and apoptotic mediators contribute significantly to the pathophysiology of all 3 components in sepsis.[2] For patients with global tissue hypoxia, as shown by increased lactate levels or hypotension, mortality can range from 36% to 46.5%.[3–6] In addition to global circulatory function, organ and microcirculatory function should also be addressed.[7] Early identification and management of threats to physiologic equilibrium, preferably before instability is clinically apparent, may prevent untoward patient outcomes.

In recent years, advances in hemodynamic monitoring have ushered the concept of physiologic signatures, specific physiologic profiles describing a disease process through time. Such profiles are constructed using an expanded set of physiologic variables and can be used to identify and manage critical illness in a timely manner. In this article, many of the physiologic variables available in current clinical practice, the successes and challenges of protocolized care that use many of these physiologic variables (goal-oriented therapy), as well as ways to address some of those challenges by building physiologic signatures are summarized. The substrate for these signatures is created through the use of a data hierarchy (**Table 1**), or the idea that new variables can be created from existing clinical variables collected at different frequencies. The goal of signature creation would be to identify a patient's location on the spectrum of critical illness and continuously assess the response to therapy.

DIAGNOSIS AND MANAGEMENT OF CRITICAL ILLNESS THROUGH CONTEMPORARY MONITORING IS GOOD, BUT CAN BE IMPROVED
Cardiopulmonary Parameters Used in Clinical Practice

Many simple variables are available to assess cardiopulmonary function and the balance between global oxygen supply and demand, but they may be nonspecific or late markers of cardiopulmonary compromise. Blood pressure is a primary determinant of

Table 1
Levels of data hierarchy

Data Hierarchy	Examples	Notes
Primary variables	HR, MAP, CVP, Scvo$_2$, SV, Spo$_2$	Used most frequently in goal-oriented therapy protocols
Secondary (derived) variables	HRV measures,[a] PPV, SVV	Requires high-frequency data collection Increasingly being integrated into goal-oriented therapy protocols
Advanced waveform analyses	Morphologic changes,[b] harmonic analyses[b]	Requires data collection via waveforms ($\geq$100 Hz) Can be performed on any variable derived from a waveform (eg, CVP, ABP)

Abbreviations: ABP, arterial blood pressure; CVP, central venous pressure; HR, heart rate; HRV, heart rate variability; MAP, mean arterial pressure; PPV, pulse pressure variability; Scvo$_2$, central venous oxygen saturation; Spo$_2$, arterial oxygen saturation measured by pulse oximetry; SV, stroke volume; SVV, stroke volume variation.
[a] The term HRV measures represents dozens of independent variables.
[b] Represent potentially hundreds of variables.

organ blood flow[8] and also provides some insight into cardiac afterload. Combined with other traditional vital signs such as heart rate (a measure of sympathetic response to physiologic stress[7]), clinicians can obtain an overall sense of cardiopulmonary health via noninvasive variables. Tachycardia is the most sensitive of all vital signs for detecting hemodynamic anomalies, but it is nonspecific and may not be present until 15% of blood volume is lost.[9]

In addition to traditional vital signs, many more reliable variables that were once only measurable through invasive devices have become available in less invasive ones. These parameters, many of them highlighted in **Table 2**, can serve to complement simple vital signs. Cardiac output is a measure of global blood flow, and therefore systemic oxygen delivery. Cardiac output changes to match metabolic demands.[7] Because cardiac output normally varies with changing end organ requirements, cardiac output measurements must be interpreted in context. One must know the changes in tissue oxygen extraction to obtain a more complete picture of the balance between metabolic need and demand. The central venous oxygen saturation ($Scvo_2$) is a minimally invasive metric used to quantify this balance. An increase in $Scvo_2$ after volume expansion reflects volume responsiveness.[10]

Some surrogate markers that are commonly used to provide hemodynamic information may be inadequate. For instance, central venous pressure (CVP) is often used as a surrogate for cardiovascular preload. However, CVP is the back-pressure to, and not a synonym for, venous return.[8] Independent of the volume of blood returning to the right heart, factors intrinsic to cardiac performance and structure can influence CVP. It is therefore not surprising that CVP is a poor marker for circulating blood volume and volume responsiveness.[11-13]

Other variables are used in clinical practice to quantify global metabolic demands. One multicenter study[14] showed that lactate clearance of 10% of the initial value was as effective as $Scvo_2$ in the protocolized resuscitation of patients during early septic shock. Central venous-to-arterial partial pressure difference of carbon dioxide (ΔPco_2) is another useful measure for determining hemodynamic status. According to the Fick principle, changes in ΔPco_2 are inversely related to changes in CO, if we assume constant total body CO_2 production. The addition of ΔPco_2 to $Scvo_2$ may predict outcome in patients with septic shock better than $Scvo_2$ alone.[15,16]

Early Detection of Cardiopulmonary Instability in Contemporary Practice Through Static Variables

Early detection of critical illness through the use of isolated hemodynamic and laboratory-based measures can be a first step toward improving outcome in patients at risk for, or those experiencing, cardiopulmonary decompensation.

- One observational study reported that patients who developed shock later than 48 hours after hospital admission had a 15.6% higher mortality in the intensive care unit (ICU) compared with those who developed shock within 48 hours of admission.[17]
- Zhen and colleagues[18] showed that septic patients identified from the emergency department (ED) had lower inpatient mortality, less mechanical ventilation in the first 24 hours after onset of shock, and a shorter time to achieve a target $Scvo_2$ than those identified later.

In the early stages of cardiopulmonary instability, before the development of hypotension or respiratory failure, clinicians may be uncertain about the presence of abnormal physiology. Generally, the triggers to initiate therapeutic interventions are crude; often using some combination of static vital signs and laboratory tests indicates

Table 2
Abbreviated list of available primary physiologic parameters

Physiologic Parameter	Interpretation	Device Used to Obtain Measurement	Level of Invasiveness
HR	Sympathetic tone	ECG monitor	Noninvasive
SBP DBP MAP PP	Sympathetic tone, cardiac contractility, vasomotor tone, and volume status	Sphygmomanometry, finger plethysmography, or arterial catheter	Noninvasive or minimally invasive[a]
SPAP DPAP MPAP PAPP	Pulmonary vascular tone, right heart contractility, and volume status	Pulmonary artery catheter	Highly invasive
P_{ra} or CVP P_{pao}[b]	Preload (static measures)	Central venous catheter or pulmonary artery catheter	Minimally invasive or highly invasive[c]
SV CO	Cardiac contractility	Finger plethysmograph,[d] arterial catheter,[d] thoracic bioimpedence, pulmonary artery catheter, and so forth	Noninvasive, minimally invasive, or highly invasive[c]
Spo_2	Arterial oxygenation	Pulse oximetry	Noninvasive
Svo_2	Total body oxygen extraction[e]	Pulmonary artery catheter	Highly invasive
Arterial pH Pao_2 Sao_2 Pco_2 Hemoglobin	Arterial oxygenation and carrying capacity	Arterial blood gas analysis[f]	Minimally invasive

Central venous pH $pcvo_2$ $Scvo_2$ $pcVco_2$	Approximate total body oxygen extraction and delivery, and metabolic clearance[e,g]	Central venous catheter	Minimally invasive
Central venous pH pvo_2 Svo_2 $pvco_2$	Total body oxygen extraction and delivery, and metabolic clearance[e]	Pulmonary artery catheter	Highly invasive
$petco_2$ Vco_2	Cardiac contractility[h]	Capnograph	Noninvasive
Global Do_2 Global Vo_2	Global oxygen delivery Global oxygen consumption	Pulmonary artery catheter	Highly invasive

Abbreviations: CO, cardiac output; CVP, central venous pressure; DBP, diastolic blood pressure; DPAP, diastolic pulmonary artery pressure; ECG, electrocardiogram; HR, heart rate; MAP, mean arterial pressure; MPAP, mean pulmonary artery pressure; Pao_2, partial pressure of oxygen; PAPP, pulmonary artery pulse pressure; Pco_2, partial pressure of carbon dioxide; $pcvo_2$, partial pressure of central venous carbon dioxide; $pcvo_2$, partial pressure of central venous oxygen; $petco_2$, end-tidal partial pressure of carbon dioxide; PP, pulse pressure; P_{pao}, pulmonary artery occlusion pressure; Pra, right atrial pressure; $pvco_2$, partial pressure of mixed venous carbon dioxide; pvo_2, partial pressure of mixed venous oxygen; Sao_2, arterial oxygen saturation; SBP, systolic blood pressure; $Scvo_2$, central venous oxygen saturation; SPAP, systolic pulmonary artery pressure; Spo_2, arterial oxygen saturation measured by pulse oximetry; SV, stroke volume; Svo_2, mixed venous oxygen saturation; Vco_2, volume of exhaled carbon dioxide.

  [a] Noninvasive if obtained from sphygmomanometry and minimally invasive if from arterial catheter.

  [b] P_{pao} is obtained from a pulmonary artery catheter only.

  [c] Noninvasive if measured by thoracic bioimpedence or finger cuff, minimally invasive if obtained from central venous catheter or arterial catheter; highly invasive if from pulmonary artery catheter or esophageal Doppler (latter not mentioned in table).

  [d] Any measures of SV or CO obtained from the finger plethysmograph or arterial catheter are from approximate calculations from arterial pressure waveform analysis. These measurements can be made only by attaching an additional monitoring device to the arterial catheter.

  [e] Oxygen delivery (and CO_2 production/clearance) can be calculated as the difference in arterial and mixed/central venous values ($\Delta pvco_2$).

  [f] From arterial vessel puncture or an arterial catheter.

  [g] Central venous values take into account only the metabolic activity of the upper body, but the differences between them and their mixed venous counterparts is marginal.

  [h] $petco_2$ and Vo_2 used as a surrogate for CO.

global tissue hypoperfusion such as lactate. These methods lack sensitivity for detecting cardiopulmonary instability at its early stages. However, these methods have proved moderately successful in clinical practice.

- Observational studies have shown that patients with trauma with increased base deficit, and strong ion difference (both measures of abnormal tissue perfusion) were most correlated with mortality.[19,20] Neither lactate[20] nor lactate clearance[21] has been shown to be predictive of outcomes in patients with trauma.
- Measures of exhaled CO_2 such as end-tidal CO_2 (petco$_2$) and volume of exhaled CO_2 (Vco$_2$) can be used as surrogate measures of CO because of their dependence on pulmonary capillary blood flow. Young and colleagues[22] showed that petco$_2$ and Vco$_2$ were both associated with volume responsiveness in patients with shock if they had no baseline lung disease. Furthermore, Dunham and colleagues[23] showed that low petco$_2$ was correlated with low CO in trauma and was therefore associated with higher injury severity scores, hypotension, major blood loss, and death.

Early Goal-Oriented Therapies: the Current Gold Standard for Dynamic Cardiopulmonary Assessment and Optimization

Goal-oriented therapeutic strategies are systematic approaches to the identification and management of cardiopulmonary decompensation that ensure the use of dynamic physiologic assessment and reassessment. Although it is important to identify impending or obvious cardiopulmonary compromise early with instantaneously measured variables, it is crucial to follow the effects of therapy with repeated measures of these variables. Early identification of impending critical illness does not itself have an effect on outcome unless it is tied to therapeutic interventions that affect outcome.[7] In applying these strategies, one must know whether they are providing the desired effect(s), or if the management strategy should be changed. Goal-oriented therapies encompass a group of proven, widely applied management strategies, which use physiologic data to not only identify pathology early but to track disease and its response to therapy over time.

Goal-oriented therapies are often multistep strategies that combine the information gained from physiologic variables obtained by noninvasive and minimally invasive means (see **Table 2**) to optimize cardiopulmonary performance. It has become important in many areas of medical practice.[3,24–32] They have proved useful for several reasons: (1) most studies assessing the use of goal-oriented therapies highlight the need to correct cardiopulmonary collapse early to minimize end organ injury and ischemia[3,24–29,31,32]; (2) goal-oriented approaches provide clear targets for resuscitation, with the intention of avoiding many of the complications, morbidity, and mortality of excessive resuscitation; and (3) goal-oriented approaches often prioritize the most important physiologic problem to correct at any given moment, with the aim of focusing clinician resources.

Goal-oriented approaches to therapy, when applied as early as possible in the disease course, positively affect outcome:

- Recent meta-analyses reported that goal-oriented approaches implemented preoperatively or perioperatively decreased the likelihood of complications in both cardiac[24,26] and noncardiac surgeries[33–35] using a range of physiologic variables.
- Other meta-analyses showed that perioperative hemodynamic optimization through use of parameter targets decreased postoperative gastrointestinal and renal dysfunction.[25,36] The benefits to renal function were seen among the

highest-risk surgical patients. Moreover, when patients were stratified by the therapeutic strategy design (fluids and inotropes versus fluids alone), the benefit of goal-oriented therapy on postoperative renal function was statistically significant only with the fluids and inotropes strategy.

- Dalfino and colleagues[37] showed in another meta-analysis that early goal-oriented therapy based on flow parameters such as cardiac output decreased the risk of postoperative infections, including pneumonia, urinary tract infections, and surgical site infections.
- A few studies have shown that goal-oriented therapies decrease perioperative wound healing and length of stay.[27,38,39]
- Rivers and colleagues[3] reported a 16% absolute risk reduction (ARR) in mortality (relative risk reduction [RRR] 34%) when early goal-directed therapy (EGDT) was applied to patients with severe sepsis and septic shock. Their approach targeted the problems of hypovolemia, vasomotor tone, oxygen carrying capacity, and cardiac dysfunction, which can be present in the septic population.
- EGDT and its dynamic use of physiologic variables is a key component of many so-called sepsis bundles, which have revolutionized care of patients with severe sepsis/septic shock. Sepsis bundles involve the protocolization of every aspect of sepsis management, including not just hemodynamic optimization but also (early) antibiotic administration. One meta-analysis[40] showed that early implementation of sepsis bundles can decrease morbidity and mortality in patients with severe sepsis and septic shock. Early hemodynamic optimization is the most important feature in bundles to improve patient outcome.[41] Early hemodynamic optimization received some of the highest recommendations in the most recent edition of the *Surviving Sepsis Campaign Guidelines*.[4]

After a patient is identified as being at risk for, or is experiencing, cardiopulmonary decompensation, therapeutic interventions used to correct the problem can lead to further problems if performed in excess.

- One study[42] showed an association between positive fluid balance and mortality in postoperative noncardiac surgery patients.
- Among patients enrolled in VASST (Vasopressin in Septic Shock Trial), those with the highest fluid balance after volume resuscitation had the highest adjusted mortality, particularly in those who had impairment in abdominal visceral perfusion secondary to profound volume overload.[43]
- A few studies have shown that a restrictive goal-oriented fluid management strategy decreased postoperative complications when compared with a more liberal approach.[44,45]
- Hayes and colleagues[46] reported that goal-oriented care in critically ill patients using supranormal targets of oxygen delivery caused an absolute risk increase in mortality of 19% in the treatment group.

The aim of any goal-oriented approach to therapy should be to resuscitate only to what is physiologically necessary. The end points of resuscitation can be defined in several ways. One approach is to use prespecified hard targets for physiologic variables without regard for individual metabolic demand. One example of this strategy is a fluid resuscitation strategy that targets only a prespecified CVP range. Although this approach may streamline the process and allow for broad, easy implementation of a goal-oriented resuscitation strategy, it may lead to either overresuscitation or underresuscitation, depending on a patient's other underlying disease(s). A better, more common approach in goal-oriented care is to: (1) correct oxygen debt, as determined by the reversal of lactic acidosis or base deficit; and (2) match metabolic supply with demand using cardiac output or $Scvo_2$, and clinical markers of end organ perfusion such as urine output and mental status assessment. This practice is highlighted in several goal-oriented approaches with proven usefulness in clinical practice.[3,30,47]

If multiple physiologic issues contribute to clinical decline, goal-oriented approaches streamline the management strategy for ease of execution. For instance, EGDT in the management of septic patients is designed to first reverse decreased organ perfusion and global tissue hypoxia by addressing hypovolemia. Once volume status is optimized (as determined by appropriate increase in CVP to a prespecified target range), vaso-motor tone is increased using vasopressors to a target mean arterial pressure. If there are still signs of oxygen supply-demand mismatch, as shown by a $Scvo_2$ less than 70%, only then is the patient transfused or given inotropes to increase oxygen delivery to tissues.[3]

Although an ordered approach of therapy allows for easy execution of resuscitation and efficient mobilization of resources, it may not represent an optimal strategy. Many of the goal-oriented approaches we have discussed collect continuous beat-to-beat data. When data are collected at this frequency, clinicians can exploit interactions be-tween physiologic variables that could be used to identify impending cardiopulmonary instability. These variable interactions could not have been used if abnormalities in physiologic variables are addressed sequentially. If high-frequency data are used in new and innovative ways, taking advantage of intervariable (and thus interorgan) inter-action, clinicians may discover new derived variables from these interactions that could be incorporated into physiologic signatures of critical illness.

TOWARD AN EARLIER DIAGNOSIS OF CARDIOPULMONARY COLLAPSE: DERIVED VARIABLES FROM HIGH-FREQUENCY CONTINUOUS DATA

Until now, only the use of primary variables has been discussed, the first level in the physiologic data hierarchy (see **Table 1**). If these variables are collected at high fre-quency, then derived variables can be constructed to aid in earlier, more accurate diagnosis of cardiopulmonary collapse (**Table 3**).

Variability Analysis

Organ cross-talk constantly takes place between multiple organs along anatomic, neural, and endocrine channels.[48] This interaction of organs forms a highly structured and tightly regulated system, which on the surface seems chaotic in view of the various physical and time scales involved but serves to couple organs for more effi-cient function of the entire organism.[49,50]

When the body encounters a disease process that acts as a systemic stressor, communication between organs, and consequently variability in organ system readout (as measured using a set of primary and secondary physiologic signals) decreases considerably or ceases altogether.[49,51] Saturation phenomena in autonomic response are the most commonly proposed explanation for decreased variability in critical illness,[52–55] but there could be additional explanations from other aspects of organ interaction manifested at different time scales. Heart rate variability (HRV) is a well-known domain comprising many secondary variables that describe various aspects of the beat-to-beat interval time series. Because beat-to-beat intervals can be acquired from any monitor that provides continuous heart rate measurements, the computation of all of these secondary variables is easily implemented at the bedside if one has the appropriate computer software.[56]

Table 3
Derived (secondary) variables and their source data

Derived Variables	Type	Source/Primary Data	Calculation
PPV	Arterial pressure variation	Pulse pressure[a]	$(PP_{max} - PP_{min})/[(PP_{max} - PP_{min}) \times 0.5]$
SVV	Arterial pressure variation	SV	$(SV_{max} - SV_{min})/SV_{mean}$
SPV	Arterial pressure variation	SBP	$SBP_{max} - SBP_{min}$ $SBP_{exp} - SBP_{min}$[b]
ΔPOP	Plethysmographic variation	Pulse oximeter waveform[c]	$(POP_{max} - POP_{min})/[(POP_{max} - POP_{min}) \times 0.5]$
PVI	Plethysmographic variation	Pulse oximeter waveform[c]	$[(PI_{max} - PI_{min})/PI_{max}] \times 100$
HRV	Variability analysis	ECG R-R interval	Variable
RRV	Variability analysis	Respiratory rate	Variable
BPV	Variability analysis	SBP, DBP, MAP	Variable
Temperature variability	Variability analysis	Continuous temperature	Variable
Glucose variability	Variability analysis	Continuous blood glucose	Variable
Waveform features	Advanced waveform analysis	Variable	Variable

Abbreviations: ΔPOP, pulse oximeter plethysmographic waveform amplitude; BPV, blood pressure variability; DBP, diastolic blood pressure; ECG, electrocardiogram; HRV, heart rate variability; MAP, mean arterial pressure; PI_{max}, maximum pleth variability index value over 1 respiratory cycle; PI_{min}, minimum pleth variability index value over 1 respiratory cycle; POP_{max}, maximum pulse oximeter plethysmographic amplitude; POP_{min}, minimum pulse oximeter plethysmographic amplitude; PP_{max}, maximum pulse pressure over a single respiratory cycle; PP_{min}, minimum pulse pressure over a single respiratory cycle; PPV, pulse pressure variation; PVI, pleth variability index; RRV, respiratory rate variability; SBP, systolic blood pressure; SBP_{exp}, systolic blood pressure during an expiratory hold; SBP_{max}, maximum systolic blood pressure over a single respiratory cycle; SBP_{min}, minimum systolic blood pressure over a single respiratory cycle; SPV, systolic pressure variation; SV, stroke volume; SV_{max}, maximum stroke volume over a given time interval; SV_{mean}, mean stroke volume over a given time interval; SV_{min}, minimum stroke volume over a given time interval; SVV, stroke volume variation.

  [a] Blood pressure parameters are measured from an arterial catheter only.

  [b] This difference is also referred to as the Δdown in the literature.

  [c] Plethysmograph variation is not dependent on the raw pulse oximetry value (ie, arterial oxygen saturation). It is calculated from the relative changes in the pulse oximeter pleth waveform.

A decrease in HRV represents increased regularity in the beat-to-beat interval time series, as measured by 1 or more secondary variables of the HRV domain. The association between decreased HRV and poor outcome in cardiovascular disease has been known for decades,[57] and stimulated work in other disease processes such as sepsis[58] and trauma.[53,59]

- There is an increasing amount of literature linking reduced HRV and sepsis in adults. Chen and Kuo[60] showed in 81 ED patients with early sepsis that HRV can be a useful method to predict impending septic shock.
- A study of 15 ED patients reported that HRV decreased in all patients who decompensated.[61]
- A pilot study of 17 bone marrow transplant patients reported that a consistent decrease in HRV occurred as sepsis developed in these patients (approximately 30 hours before conventional vital signs).[62]
- Fathizadeh and colleagues[53] showed that pathologic changes in autonomic function occurred before tachycardia among a cohort of patients with trauma without severe injury.
- Increasing evidence from human data[59] and animal models[63] suggests that HRV is superior to traditional vital signs in detecting hemodynamic decompensation from trauma. Decreased HRV is associated with mortality among patients with trauma in the prehospital setting[64] and in the trauma ICU.[59]

Although the evidence linking decreased HRV and other variability analyses to clinical decompensation is increasing, there are still many challenges limiting their clinical use. Most bedside monitors do not hold in memory the continuous vitals data that are shown at a degree of granularity necessary to compute secondary variables characterizing HRV in real time. However, variability analyses can be performed in real time with appropriate software.[56] Even if one is able to perform variability analysis, HRV and respiratory rate variability (RRV) can be affected by medications such as sedatives or vasopressors. One study showed that HRV and RRV can still be reliably identified in mechanically ventilated patients on sedation.[65] HRV can be characterized by dozens of derived variables (**Table 4**) with varying degrees of correlation between these variables. There is no clear evidence showing the superiority of any HRV-related variable, and there are no guidelines as to how to obtain an overall assessment of HRV. This finding extends to variability analyses of all other primary physiologic signals, such as blood pressure, oximetry, respiratory rate, or temperature. The potential benefits of variability analysis need to be clarified and confirmed in more rigorous study in different populations at risk for clinical deterioration.

Arterial Pressure Variation and Plethysmograph Variability

When physiologic variables are collected on a beat-to-beat, or continuous basis (>100 Hz), more additional variables can be computed from these primary signals. Together with the time series of primary physiologic variables, these secondary, or derived, variables could identify impending cardiopulmonary collapse earlier than the variables from which they are derived. It can be speculated that such predictive secondary variables reflect deep physiologic interactions that are perturbed early in the process of cardiovascular instability.

Variables calculated from arterial pressure variation are dynamic and therefore estimate preload dependence, the key factor in predicting volume responsiveness. Preload dependence is superior to static measures of preload such as CVP, because preload is not the only determinant of preload dependence.[66] A fluid bolus leads to an

Table 4		
HRV domain groups and an abbreviated list of derived variable examples		
Domain	**Comments**	**Variable Examples**
Statistical	Describe statistical features of time-series data; assumes the state of subsequent data is determined independent of prior data	SDNN, RMSSD, NN50, pNN50, IQRNN
Frequency	Deconstructs R-R interval sequences into their spectral components to construct the power distribution of the time series	Total power, ULF, VLF, LF, HF, LF/HF
Geometric	Identifies and creates a shape from the histogram representation of some specified property in an R-R interval series (see indices column)	NN interval length distribution, Poincare plot, differential index, TINN, HTI
Nonlinear methods	Describes properties that show fractality, and other characteristics that do not vary in time and space	SampEn, ApEn, Shannon entropy, DFA, Lyapunov exponents, dispersion analysis

Abbreviations: ApEn, approximate entropy; DFA, detrended fluctuation analysis; HF, high frequency (0.15–0.4 Hz); HTI, heart rate variability triangular index; IQRNN, interquartile range of NN; LF, low frequency (0.04–0.15 Hz); NN, the interval between 2 normal R-waves (ie, from nonectopic beats); NN50, number of interval differences of successive NN intervals >50 ms; pNN50, proportion derived by dividing NN50 by the total NN intervals; RMSSD, squared root of the mean squared differences of successive; R-R, interval between peaks of two consecutive R-waves, irrespective of whether the heart beats are normal or not; SampEn, sample entropy; SDNN, the standard deviation of all NN intervals; TINN, triangular interpolation of NN interval histogram; ULF, ultralow frequency (≤0.003 Hz); VLF, very low range (0.003–0.04 Hz).

increase in cardiac output only if: (1) the patient has good baseline cardiac function; and (2) the patient's cardiovascular status places them on the steep, or preload-dependent portion of the Frank-Starling curve. Volume responsiveness is best estimated with dynamic assessment of physiologic variables collected at high frequency.

Measures of arterial pressure variation (namely pulse pressure variation [PPV], systolic pressure variation [SPV], and stroke volume variation [SVV]) use the normal changes that occur in the arterial waveform during mechanical ventilation to assess hypovolemia. Early in a positive pressure breath, the increase in intrathoracic pressure causes compression of pulmonary veins. This process leads to an increase in left atrial pressure, and left ventricular (LV) preload. The concomitant decrease in left-sided afterload causes an increase in LV stroke volume (SV) and blood pressure. Meanwhile, the increased intrathoracic pressure decreases venous return, and thus right-sided preload and SV. Toward the end of inspiration or beginning of expiration, the lower SV from the right ventricle reaches the left heart, causing a decrease in LVSV and blood pressure.[67] This normal heart-lung interaction is exaggerated in someone who is hypovolemic.

- In 1 meta-analysis, arterial pressure variation was shown to be sensitive and specific in predicting volume responsiveness, outperforming static measures of preload such as CVP.[12] PPV seemed to perform slightly better than SVV (area under the curve [AUC] 0.94 vs 0.84, respectively).

- Michard and colleagues[68] showed that PPV of 13% or more identified volume responders with a sensitivity of 94% and specificity of 98%. Although their study was conducted on patients with rather large tidal volumes, these findings were validated in a population with acute respiratory distress syndrome showing lower tidal volumes and high positive end-expiratory pressure (PEEP).[69]
- Zhang and colleagues[70] showed in 1 meta-analysis that SVV had a diagnostic odds ratio of 18.4 to predict volume responsiveness in the operating room and ICU, with good sensitivity and specificity. The literature supports measuring SVV only in patients on a control mode ventilation with tidal volumes of 8 mL/kg or more.[70] However, many studies in this study measured SVV in patients receiving smaller tidal volumes and published AUCs of 0.8 or greater for predicting volume responsiveness. The investigators did not report the PEEP for the patients in these studies.
- Several studies have validated the use of arterial pressure variation as a marker of volume responsiveness in goal-oriented therapeutic protocols that decreased many complications, including organ failure.[33–35,71]
- Multiple studies have looked at SPV as a marker of volume of responsiveness, with conflicting results.[68,72–75] However, Tavernier and colleagues[76] showed that when systolic blood pressure (SBP) is measured during a clinician-initiated expiratory pause on the ventilator, the difference between that SBP measurement and the minimum SBP in the next respiratory cycle (termed the Δdown) can predict volume responsiveness.

Before the development of new noninvasive devices that can produce arterial tracings,[77–79] investigators have studied whether plethysmograph variation can be a noninvasive surrogate for the arterial pressure variation taken from an arterial catheter.

- Cannesson and colleagues[80] showed that changes in pulse oximetry plethysmograph tracings correlated highly with PPV.
- Forget and colleagues[31] reported lower lactate levels among patients in whom plethysmograph variation was used as a marker of volume responsiveness, compared with patients who had no dynamic measure of preload dependence.
- One meta-analysis involving 326 critically ill and perioperative patients showed that the pleth variability index (1 measure of plethysmograph variation) was able to identify preload responsive patients (diagnostic odds ratio 16.0; area under receiver operating characteristic 0.87).[81] This was particularly true among adults and those on mechanical ventilation.

The usefulness of PPV as a clinically relevant and actionable secondary variable is appealing from elementary physiologic considerations. Many more variables derived from primary signals may also be useful predictors of instability that relate to deeper, more complex, but no less important physiologic disruptions.

ADVANCED WAVEFORM ANALYSIS: UNTAPPED SECONDARY VARIABLES

PPV, SVV, and SPV are all detected via simple analyses of arterial waveforms, but there is a wealth of information that could be gathered from more sophisticated analyses of digitized waveform data. Physiologic waveforms contain information collected at a higher frequency than is available from intervals (such as the R-R interval in HRV). There is potential to uncover more about impending cardiopulmonary decompensation than what could be gathered from beat-to-beat-dependent variables. It is thus at the highest level in the data hierarchy constructed to create physiologic signatures of critical illness (see **Table 1**). Moreover, it is possible to extract important information not only from arterial waveforms (as is already available clinically through arterial pressure variation) but also from CVP and other waveforms that are currently underused. The information collected from these secondary signals could play a key role in the construction of physiologic signatures.

One straightforward, yet potentially productive approach is to track changes in the morphology of waveforms. All physiologic waveforms have a characteristic shape for 1 normal cycle. Certain disease processes cause changes to the shape of these waveforms, which, although not pathognomonic, can identify the presence of disease.[67,82] For instance, cardiac tamponade is 1 well-known cause of the pulsus paradoxus pattern in the arterial waveform, which morphologically is distinct from the normal shape and structure of the arterial wave. Similarly, in the presence of an atrial arrhythmia or tricuspid regurgitation, the CVP waveform also undergoes changes from its normal morphology.[67] In contemporary practice, the CVP waveform is used simply to extract the CVP value at end expiration.[83] With the appropriate technology,[83] other secondary variables can be extracted from CVP that could be used to predict cardiopulmonary decompensation by expressing the underlying physiology.

- Roy and colleagues[84] showed that it is possible to measure the difference in size of the wave components in 1 cycle of CVP through time. Although these investigators found no difference between fluid responders and nonresponders, they did not look at how these wave components change in size with time, potentially providing additional key information.

A more complicated, but more comprehensive, approach for morphologic analysis and secondary predictor extraction from waveforms is to use harmonic analysis. This approach breaks a waveform down into a superposition of sinusoidal waves of decreasing wavelengths, which in turn undergo signal processing to extract useful information. Fourier transform (FT) is the most commonly used signal processing approach performed on physiologic waveforms.[85] FT yields a power spectrum, a summary of the contribution of sine waves of varying frequencies to the original waveform. The goal in advanced waveform analysis is to detect changes in the underlying physiology over time. FT requires additional modifications to be applied on dynamically changing waveforms, and therefore it is more useful to use a signal processing approach that inherently takes this into account.

Wavelet analysis incorporates the temporal evolution of a signal, potentially allowing one to better identify physiologic decompensation. De Melis and colleagues[86] have shown that it is possible to implement these transforms on arterial pressure waveform data. Wavelet transform offers the added advantage of analyzing time windows of different lengths.[86]

THE CHALLENGE OF DATA GRANULARITY

Any tool used to create physiologic signatures of critical illness should retrieve the most meaningful variables at a specific point in disease progression and present them to clinicians to inform decision making. For instance, if PPV and SVV are increased (indicating volume responsiveness) in a patient who is at risk for pneumonia, this may indicate the early stages of sepsis (simple hypovolemia). However, if a clinician encounters the same patient with a high PPV and SVV, abnormal variables extracted from the CVP waveform, low CO, and some of the HRV variables are decreased indicating some aberrancy in autonomic tone, then this patient may be much further along the disease process. The physiologic signature of the former state may even be able to predict when the latter state would occur.

There are several potential variables at different data hierarchy levels that could be incorporated into a physiologic signature at any given point in the evolution of a disease process (see **Table 1**). **Tables 2** and **3** review some variables that are already used in contemporary practice. If the dozens of available variability variables are added to that (see **Table 4**), and the hundreds of variables that could be extracted from each waveform, it would be impossible for a busy bedside clinician to manually synthesize all of these potentially useful data to find those that are abnormal, and then make decisions about where patients are in the critical illness spectrum.[87]

The challenge of data granularity (the density of information that can be used in a prediction model) is shown in **Fig. 1**. The top of the figure represents raw data (as outlined in **Table 2**) collected at different frequencies (some intermittent, and some waveform data). As more secondary variables are extrapolated from the primary signals (see **Table 2** and variables from advanced waveform analyses), the data granularity increases. When critical mass is reached (represented by the bottom of **Fig. 1**), there are hundreds, if not thousands, of secondary variables. How does one process all of these data to retrieve meaningful information to construct physiologic signatures of critical illness? Several existing approaches used to create physiologic signatures for early diagnosis and therapeutic management of critical illness are summarized.

CREATING PHYSIOLOGIC SIGNATURES OF CRITICAL ILLNESS USING MACHINE LEARNING

Machine learning refers to a rich discipline in computer science dedicated to the design and implementation of automated computer-based methods and algorithms to identify patterns in typically large data sets. Standard statistical analysis such as logistic regression can be construed as a subset of those methods. The application

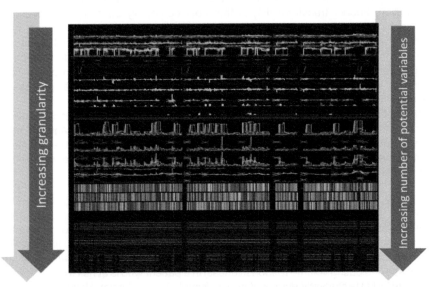

Fig. 1. Data granularity. How data granularity can dramatically increase with secondary variable derivation. The top of this diagram shows approximately 1.5 patient-years of data. Because derived variables are extracted from primary parameters (intermittent, continuous, and waveform data), there is a remarkable increase in data granularity. The bottom of the figure represents greater than 7000 variables (more than the amount of pixels needed to show all of them on a screen).

of a machine learning approach can efficiently deal with densely granular data. Although there are many different approaches that could be used (**Table 5**), there is a common process that can be applied to the identification of physiologic signatures in critical illness as depicted in **Fig. 2**:

- Any machine learning approach has to generate models that are generalizable, and therefore, learning must proceed on a patient cohort of a sufficient size as to include several instances of signatures representative of disease evolution. The learned signatures are disease process specific.
- All primary, secondary variables, and extracted variables from waveforms are obtained or computed from the primary patient data.
- All variables in the data hierarchy (see **Table 1**) are used as input to machine learning algorithms. Different machine learning approaches have different tools for classifying and predicting. The algorithms generate models that offer a prediction given primary data. The nature of the prediction depends on the learning task. A typical learning task relevant to the identification of clinically applicable physiologic signatures is to estimate a normal trajectory of predictor variables and classify a new case as abnormal if 1 or more predictors deviate from that trajectory.[88]
- Because it is not necessary, and would likely be inefficient, for the model to use all data for accurate classification, the algorithm chooses the most informative features at a particular point in time in the disease process.
- A set of algorithms are applied to maximize external validity of the predictions.
- In a typical application, the model is applied to data from a test case, continuously updated as data accrue, and generates an instantaneous predictive forecast of what is expected to happen over a specified time horizon.
- More patients and their data could then be added to the derivation/validation cohorts for model refinement.

Static forms of machine learning algorithms have already been applied in many fields, including weather forecasting[89] and infectious disease biosurveillance.[90] It has also been applied in medicine.[91–94] Machine learning is applicable to a broad scope of acute care settings, including ED triage,[95] and the ICU.[96,97] It is also applicable to specific diseases like sepsis[98–101] and traumatic hemorrhage.[93,98,102–104] Applications of machine learning to learn physiologic signatures represent a step forward from static classifications and predictions, in that it is dynamic in nature; predictions are updated, and models can potentially continue to learn adaptively as data are accrued.

The machine learning approach has a few advantages: first, machine learning can use all available physiologic data (primary data collected intermittently or continuously) and variables derived from beat-to-beat data (eg, PPV, SVV, HRV) and advanced waveform features. Second, once a subject is classified, a model can show other aspects of the disease process, such as the amount of fluid/blood that was lost. Glass and colleagues[105] were able to identify not only bleeding, but the amount of blood lost under experimental conditions of controlled hemorrhage in an animal model using machine learning. The same findings were confirmed in simulated hemorrhage in patients using lower body negative pressure (LBNP) to reduce central blood volume.[106] This factor would be critical to an approach used to identify the physiologic signatures at all points in the evolution of impending critical illness. Third, many algorithms deal effectively with correlated or missing data. Model building through machine learning is an iterative process. New patient data are incorporated into older versions of the model to refine prediction. Model building from machine

Table 5
Some commonly used machine learning techniques

Technique	Overview	Comments
Regression analysis	Determines the probable expectation of a dependent variable based on training data from an independent variable(s) in a subject sample. Dependent variables can be dichotomous or continuous, depending on the type of regression.	Every type of regression has assumptions, for instance, about linear/nonlinear relationships between dependent and independent variables. Care must be taken to know these assumptions before application
Decision tree learning	Uses decision trees to classify data. Algorithm determines the most informative attribute given a set of observations, and splits the data set according to this attribute (divide-and-conquer algorithm). Process repeated recursively.	Overfitting is common; prevented by pruning algorithms
Support vector machine (SVM)	Based on linear optimization; subjects are classified in a way that maximizes the distance between the observations and a separation hyperplane (hyperplane margin).	
k-Nearest neighbor (kNN)	Given an unlabeled (test) observation, kNN looks for the k most similar observations in the training cohort. k and the definition of similarity are defined by the user. The most represented class of labeled observations from the training cohort is the output	Relatively simple to construct
k-means clustering	Iterative process used to partition data into k clusters. Clusters initiated by picking k centroids, or cluster focal points. Iteration involves assigning new data points to the closest centroid (closeness is user defined), then reweighting each cluster mean to the geometric center of the new cluster.	Simple to understand and execute. Sensitive to initiation and therefore may change with every execution. Algorithm may fail if clusters are not distinct when the process is complete. Optimal k often tested by trial and error
Artificial neural networks (ANN)	Models simulate brain organization. Neurons (nodes) receive weighted inputs, and output a transfer function. Groups of these building blocks form a network. Training data adjust input weights and build/destroy connections.	Show complex/nonlinear behavior based on the connection network. Can be used for supervised (involving experts) or unsupervised (automated) learning
Ensemble learning algorithms	Learns sets of classifiers and merges their outputs. Classifiers are trained independently on specific sets of training observations. In boosting, each subsequent training set emphasizes importance of training samples that have been problematic for the models that are already part of the ensemble. Some ensembles (eg, Random Forest) use a bagging (bootstrap aggregation) approach. Separate decision trees are learned from independent samples of the training data. Multiple random samples (of subjects or attributes) yield the ensemble of models.	Robust; can handle small number of samples

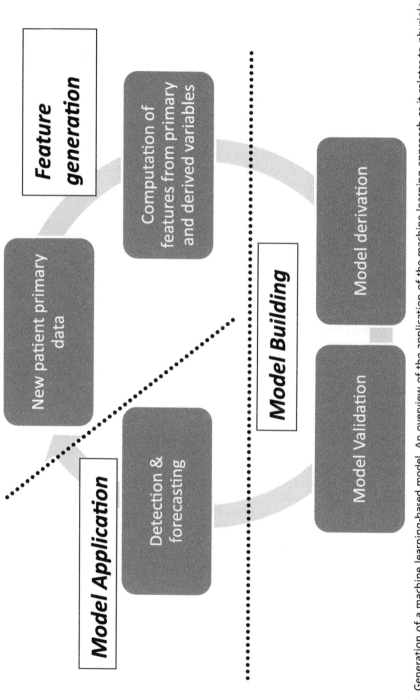

Fig. 2. Generation of a machine learning-based model. An overview of the application of the machine learning approach as it relates to physiologic signature generation. New patient data are featurized to create input from physiologic variables. The model is derived and internally validated on a cohort of training data. It is then applied to a test case for the detection and prediction of clinical instability. New data may be added to the training set to refine model performance.

learning represents best clinical practice; clinicians identify and treat disease more effectively when they encounter more patients with the disease.

Machine learning algorithms are used by several existing models in critical illness prediction. Many models build fused parameters, which function as an effective simplification of multiparameter physiologic signatures. Fused parameters incorporate multiple data inputs and integrate them to form a single value used in decision making. Three such parameters from the literature are highlighted.

The Visensia Stability Index

The Visensia Stability Index (VSI) is a fused parameter built by the Visensia software (OBS Medical, Oxford, UK) designed as an integrated monitoring tool. Visensia automatically processes and integrates simple noninvasively measured vital sign data in real time. It converts multiparameter monitoring into a single parameter for interpretation by health care professionals (**Fig. 3**).

Development of the VSI is data driven and specific to the patient population. Unlike many of the existing goal-directed strategies for early identification of critical illness discussed in previous sections, Visensia does not depend on an artificial cutoff of vital signs for abnormality. Instead, it uses k-means clustering (see **Table 5**), which is trained on a robust cohort of similar patients before the VSI is used for decision-making purposes. It identifies normality and then quantifies departures from this, and an alert is triggered if 1 vital sign is ±3 standard deviations (SD) from normal, or if 2 or more vital signs are outside normal range by a smaller amount.[107] The appropriate cutoff value for the VSI is determined from the training data set based on these training-specific norms. An alert is triggered when the VSI value goes over this cutoff for 80% of the time in a time window of a set length. The major strength of the algorithm is that it triggers an alert before patients show signs of obvious abnormality such as hypotension.

There are 2 major studies that have discussed the VSI and its role in instability identification:

- Watkinson and colleagues[108] randomized 402 high-risk medical and surgical ward patients to usual monitoring versus VSI monitoring. Their primary outcome was the proportion of patients experiencing major adverse events, including the activation of a rapid response service, transfer to an ICU, and mortality. They found no difference in these outcomes between the 2 groups. The study design did not institute a protocol to address an emergency if one arose, so no intervention was tied to the monitoring. Moreover, many patients in the control arm had multiparameter monitoring (eg, an electrocardiography [ECG] monitor and pulse oximeter). There was likely contamination of the control group if clinicians recognized instability that the VSI also would have recognized.
- Hravnak and colleagues[109] studied the difference in the incidence of cardiopulmonary instability before and after implementation of the Visensia system in a stepdown unit population. They found that the number of alerts decreased by 58%, and the amount of time patients spent with unstable vital signs decreased by 60%. The number of instability episodes (defined by the local medical emergency team (MET) protocol and not the VSI) decreased by 70%. In those patients with both VSI alerts and unstable vitals (again defined by the local MET), the VSI alert preceded the unstable vital sign by an average of 9 minutes.

Survival Probability

Bayard and colleagues devised a search and display, or stochastic, program, which outputs a survival probability (SP). The SP is another fused parameter

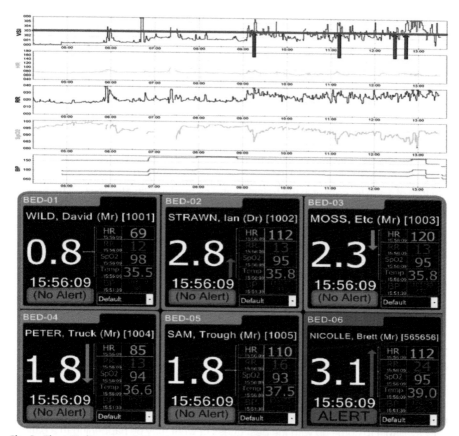

Fig. 3. The VSI. (*Top panel*) The time series of a modified VSI (without temperature) used in 1 academic center is shown for 1 stepdown unit patient, alongside the vital sign components of the VSI. A VSI of 3.2 (*red line*) was the cutoff value selected based on a training data set of a similar patient population. If the VSI was consistently higher than this value, the alert would be triggered (*red arrows*) and would stay activated as long as the VSI stayed more than 3.2 (*red portions of VSI tracing*). A medical emergency team (MET) was called to see this patient at 13:29; the VSI alert was triggered 4 times beforehand based often on subtle changes in 1 or more vital signs. (The first alert was more than 4 hours before the MET activation.) (*Bottom panel*) A monitor showing the VSI and its component vitals from multiple patients simultaneously. The monitor shows not only the current VSI value for a given patient, but the trend based on previous values. (The cutoff value in this patient population was 3.0.) (*Courtesy of* OBS Medical; with permission.)

derived from a probabilistic model that integrates several physiologic predictors representative of global (CO, Spo_2) and regional perfusion (transcutaneous oxygen and CO_2 tensions).

Similar to the VSI, the SP is derived from a training set of patients with similar clinical and physiologic states, defined by their primary diagnoses, comorbidities, and hemodynamics, among other factors. The machine learning approach of choice was k nearest neighbors (see **Table 5**). The algorithm looks at 40 or more similar nearest neighbor states, and predicts survival of a test case based on these training set examples.

- When the SP system was applied to a cohort of 396 severely ill patients with trauma, the SP was 25% lower among nonsurvivors compared with survivors.[110] It accurately classified survivors and nonsurvivors 91.4% of the time.

Unlike the VSI, there is a decision-support component built into the system that creates the SP. One can quantify the relative efficiency of a therapy used in the nearest neighbors case to inform decision making.[111]

Compensatory Reserve Index

The compensatory reserve index (CRI) was devised to identify acute volume loss. It is a fused parameter calculated from waveform analysis, SV, SpO_2, $petCO_2$, along with vital sign data. The CRI is calculated by comparing the patient's arterial waveform features with that of a similar patient in the training set. The model estimates the CRI for a given patient based on the CRI value of those in the training set with similar input features.

- Convertino and colleagues[112] assessed if the CRI was able to identify persons with low stressor tolerance (fainters) and high stressor tolerance (nonfainters) in 101 participants exposed to LBNP. (LBNP was used to simulate a decrease in central blood volume, and thus intravascular blood volume.) CRI was able to identify low-tolerance patients with hemodynamic decompensation when SV was not decreased. From these results, the investigators inferred that the CRI is an estimate of cardiovascular reserve.

CREATING PHYSIOLOGIC SIGNATURES OF CRITICAL ILLNESS FROM HEURISTIC MODELS: THE ROTHMAN INDEX

Fused parameters can be calculated from rule-based approaches applied on a broad scale that serve similar goals as machine learning algorithms (ie, these rule-based algorithms can select the most useful data from the wealth of information that is clinically available to come up with the best guess of what may be happening to a patient at any given moment). The Rothman index (RI) is a heuristic model that uses not only physiologic data (vital signs) but also standardized nursing assessments of organ systems, laboratory data, and cardiac rhythm information from hemodynamic monitors to construct a fused parameter. Unlike fused parameters that use machine learning, the goal is not to forecast what could happen; the goal of the RI is simply to describe a patient's current condition.[113]

According to Rothman and colleagues, the RI takes 43 continuously streaming clinical variables from a range of sources in the electronic medical records of patients and applies risk functions, or mathematical equations, to their behavior with respect to some outcome. The creators of the RI defined excess risk as a percent increase in 1-year all-cause mortality associated with a given value of a variable when compared with the minimum possible mortality of that variable. These mortality risks were determined from a derivation cohort. The goal was not to predict mortality but to use an easily determined outcome that closely correlated with discharge condition. The model was constructed by summing the excess risk input from the 26 variables that independently affected 1-year all-cause mortality; the excess risk values for each variable were subtracted from 100 to calculate the RI. The granularity of certain data sources such as laboratory values may be low. The RI controlled for that by applying smoothing functions that would scale the relative importance of data based on its age; newer values for certain variables weighted more with respect to their excess risk input compared with older values of other variables. Scores were calculated on a derivation cohort and validated in 5 separate cohorts.

The RI can identify clinical instability based on several studies:

- In a cohort of medical and surgical patients, Bradley and colleagues[114] showed that patients with highest-risk RIs (RI<70) and moderate-risk RIs (RI 70–79) had 2.65 higher odds, and 2.40 higher odds of readmission, respectively, compared with those with the lowest-risk RIs.
- Another study[115] showed that the RI, when compared with the Modified Early Warning Score (an established early warning system designed to predict impending cardiopulmonary arrest), correlated better with 24-hour mortality (receiver operating characteristic 0.82 and 0.93, respectively).
- Tepas and colleagues[116] showed that initial RI values correlated with postoperative complication rates in a cohort of surgical patients. Moreover, as complications ensued in any given patient, the RI decreased, suggesting progressive physiologic dysfunction.

The strength of the RI is that it gives a longitudinal view of patient condition with the goal of early detection of pathologic trends.

CREATING PHYSIOLOGIC SIGNATURES OF CRITICAL ILLNESS FROM HEART RATE CHARACTERISTICS: THE HERO SCORE

Some fused parameters may use a portion of the available variables that could be used to create physiologic signatures. The HeRO score is a fused parameter used to detect neonatal sepsis, a prevalent disease process in the neonatal ICU with a significant mortality reaching 20% in preterm infants.[117] The score is not derived from many components, but it is a powerful physiologic signature for identifying impending neonatal critical illness.

The HeRO score incorporates 2 common HRV variables: SD of R-R intervals from 2 nonectopic heartbeats (SDNN) and sample entropy (SampEn). (SampEn is a robust measure of the irregularity, or randomness in a time series.[118,119]) The HeRO score also incorporates information about heart rate accelerations and decelerations. Sample asymmetry refers to the relative frequency of heart rate accelerations and decelerations. Sudden transient decelerations in heart rate are pathologic phenomena of unexplained cause unique to the neonatal population, causing an increase in sample asymmetry.[118]

The HeRO score is a composite metric derived from SDNN, SampEn, and sample asymmetry. It measures the patient's probability of developing sepsis in 24 hours, normalized to the average probability of a similar patient population. It is shown as the fold-increase in probability of developing sepsis, with 1 or less being normal or low risk and 5 representing a 5-fold increased risk of developing sepsis over the next 24 hours.[118]

In the years since the creators first noted the association between transient heart rate decelerations and the clinical diagnosis of sepsis,[120] the HeRO score has proved itself to be a highly useful early detection tool in neonates:

- Griffin and colleagues[121] showed that reduced variability and transient decelerations (the latter being specific to the neonatal population) can identify culture-positive and culture-negative sepsis up to 5 days before the clinical suspicion of sepsis determined by traditional vital sign measurements.
- In the largest clinical trial of very low birth weight (VLBW) infants to date, Moorman and colleagues[122] randomized 3003 VLBW neonates to traditional monitoring versus HeRO monitoring. They found that simply providing health care providers with the HeRO monitor caused a statistically significant RRR in

mortality of 20.5% (ARR = 2.1%) among VLBW infants. Similar findings were seen in extremely low birth weight infants (RRR = 25%; ARR = 4.4%).

The HeRO score stands out as a physiologic signature of disease. Most clinical decompensation seen in neonates is caused by sepsis,[118] and the interventions are usually specific (blood culture with or without antibiotic administration). So, although there are no specific therapeutic interventions tied to early detection, it seems that the success of the score lies in its ability to draw attention to a particular patient for the initiation of those interventions. Also, clinicians using the HeRO monitor are encouraged to incorporate the HeRO score into routine clinical assessment. One study prepared a scorecard to help predict sepsis, incorporating information from the HeRO score and routinely used clinical signs. The HeRO score incrementally improved accurate prediction of sepsis in those with low risk determined from clinical evaluation.[123]

Because the HeRO score does not use the scope of all potentially useful data, there is no need for machine learning approaches in its implementation. It is constructed from 3 variables that the designers proved would provide the most valuable information in the neonatal population.[119] These variables exemplify the complex nonlinear behavior of physiology and organ-organ interaction that may be lost in the process of clinical decompensation, specifically in the development of neonatal sepsis.

CREATING PHYSIOLOGIC SIGNATURES OF CRITICAL ILLNESS FROM MULTIORGAN MONITORING

Seely and colleagues[124] describe the Continuous Individualized Multiorgan Variability Analysis (CIMVA) software as a tool designed to take multiorgan input (mainly cardiac [ECG] and respiratory [end-tidal capnography]) and perform variability analyses. The output from the system is the following: (1) a matrix of numerical results (the variability measures) organized in chronologic order of analysis windows and (2) a summary report. The creators expect that by producing these variability measures at every point in the evolution of disease, users would gain some insight into changing organ-organ dynamics, identifying new emergent properties of this complex system that would be informative.

There are preliminary studies that show the potential usefulness of a technology like CIMVA for creating physiologic signatures of critical illness:

- In a study of 33 patients, Green and colleagues[125] assessed the trajectory of CIMVA multiorgan output during the development of shock, and the resolution of respiratory failure. HRV and RRV variables started to decrease about 12 to 18 hours before the onset of shock. Patients who were successfully extubated had higher HRV measurements before and after extubation. RRV showed an upward trend beginning 10 hours before extubation indicating the resolution of disease.
- Seely and colleagues[124] assessed whether there was a correlation between multiorgan monitoring and failed extubation after a spontaneous breathing trial (SBT). Patients who failed extubation after SBT had a greater loss of certain RRV measures compared with patients who passed extubation. (Some HRV measures showed a similar reduction that was not statistically significant.)

CIMVA could constitute a feasible[65] and viable platform from which physiologic signatures can be generated.

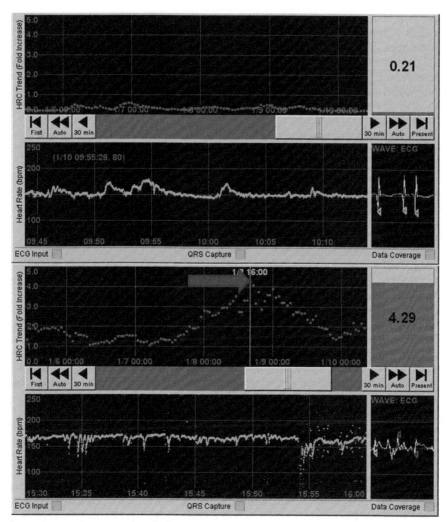

Fig. 4. Contrasting normal and abnormal patient data on the HeRO (HRC) monitor. (*Top panel*) Still photograph of patient in a neonatal ICU. The bottom half represents 30 minutes of heart rate data (*green tracing*, in beats per minute). Note the normal variation in heart rate. The top half represents 5 days of continuous HRC output, representing a fold increase in risk of sepsis over the next 24 hours (*orange tracing*). The HeRO score (HRC index) at the time was less than 1, indicating a low risk of developing sepsis. (*Bottom panel*) By contrast, a still photograph of a different patient shows a heart rate tracing with frequent decelerations. The corresponding HRC tracing has a spike (*red arrow*) corresponding to a HeRO score of 4.29. When this photograph was taken, this patient was more than 4 times more likely to develop sepsis in the next 24 hours when compared with similar patients in a control sample.

CHALLENGES TO THE GENERATION OF PHYSIOLOGIC SIGNATURES IN CRITICAL ILLNESS

The techniques described for physiologic signature creation in the critically ill are cutting edge; most have not been executed in widespread clinical practice, and none of them is considered standard of care for cardiopulmonary monitoring in any disease process. Potential challenges must be overcome before this groundbreaking research can be applied on a large scale.

Current hardware and network configurations are not readily amenable to data-intensive, third-party applications, which may need to draw from physiologic data streams and the electronic health record. Improving system interoperability is a necessary step toward the implementation of advanced physiologic monitoring tools on standard monitoring platforms.

Some clinicians and hospitals may be skeptical of using machine learning algorithms to drive identification and therapeutic management of critical illness. They may fear the application of a process that occurs, from their perspective, in a black box. Some may even believe that they are being replaced by these algorithms. However, as available data increase, it will become impossible for clinicians in a busy work environment to select the most important variables to use for medical decision making at any given time.[126] Hospitals and health care professionals will need to be in-serviced on the benefits of integrating machine learning approaches into everyday practice.

Clinicians are not accustomed to seeing physiologic data merged to form new values, making it difficult to interpret the output of numerical fused parameters derived from machine learning techniques, the RI or the HeRO score. Perhaps one way to deal with fused parameters is to provide a visual tool, an innovative way that can explain which component of the cardiopulmonary system is wrong. This strategy could provide clinicians with some structure on how to therapeutically correct the abnormalities detected. Some fused parameters already provide some graphical or diagrammatic platform,[127] including the HeRO score (**Fig. 4**) and VSI. The key is to provide the means by which clinicians can apply/change management in response to what they see. It is possible that the application of certain fused parameters did not show the expected outcomes because this was not done.[108]

SUMMARY

Physiologic data are the building blocks for the physiologic signatures of critical illness. It is the dynamic behavior of physiologic variables that makes them ideal for this purpose. The numeric value of a physiologic variable and its relation to previous measurements can identify the presence of disease and inform clinicians about a patient's current position in the evolution of a disease process. By looking at physiologic data in new ways, an increasing number of derived variables are being created from primarily measured data like CO. Derived variables, many already available for bedside use, provide additional information previously unavailable to clinicians about the physiologic behavior of certain diseases. Waveforms contain physiologic data that are grossly underused, and may be more useful than the static, intermittent values that are extracted from them. There are many ways to construct physiologic signatures from available data to identify and manage impending critical illness in a timely manner. If all data are to be used, the granularity, or density, of data will reach a point at which novel techniques of data synthesis will be essential. Machine learning approaches can be helpful for that purpose. Fused parameters can be constructed to synthesize the data into a usable format, although machine learning may not be needed if the data are not highly granular. Future study is necessary to assess the use of physiologic signatures in improving patient outcome, particularly when signature use is tied to interventions. It is clear that timely identification and management of critical illness or impending decompensation are important. Clinicians should use all available data to their full potential to reach this goal.

REFERENCES

1. Kauvar DS, Lefering R, Wade CE. Impact of hemorrhage on trauma outcome: an overview of epidemiology, clinical presentations, and therapeutic considerations. J Trauma 2006;60:S3–11.
2. Otero RM, Nguyen HB, Huang DT, et al. Early goal directed therapy in severe sepsis and septic shock revisited: concept, controversies, and contemporary findings. Chest 2006;130:1579–95.
3. Rivers EP, Nguyen B, Havstad S, et al. Early goal-directed therapy in the treatment of severe sepsis and septic shock. N Engl J Med 2001;345:1368–77.
4. Dellinger RP, Levy MM, Rhodes A, et al. Surviving sepsis campaign: international guidelines for management of severe sepsis and septic shock: 2012. Crit Care Med 2013;41:580–637.
5. Shapiro NI, Howell MD, Talmor D, et al. Serum lactate as a predictor of mortality in emergency department patients with infection. Ann Emerg Med 2005;45: 524–8.
6. Trzeciak S, Chansky ME, Dellinger RP, et al. Operationalizing the use of serum lactate measurement for identifying high risk of death in a clinical practice algorithm for suspected severe sepsis. Acad Emerg Med 2006;13(Suppl 1):S150–1.
7. Pinsky MR. Hemodynamic evaluation and monitoring in the ICU. Chest 2007; 132:2020–9.
8. Pinsky MR, Payen D. Functional hemodynamic monitoring. Crit Care 2005;9: 566–72.
9. American College of Surgeons Trauma Committee. Advanced trauma life support for doctors. 8th edition. Chicago: American College of Surgeons; 2008.
10. Giraud R, Siegenthaler N, Gayet-Ageron A, et al. ScvO2 as a marker to define fluid responsiveness. J Trauma 2011;70:802–7.
11. Kumar A, Anel R, Bunnell E, et al. Pulmonary artery occlusion pressure and central venous pressure fail to predict ventricular filling volume, cardiac performance, or the response to volume infusion in normal subjects. Crit Care Med 2004;32:691–9.
12. Marik PE, Baram M, Vahid B. Does central venous pressure predict volume responsiveness? A systematic review of the literature and the tale of seven mares. Chest 2008;134:172–8.
13. Oohashi S, Endoh H. Does central venous pressure or pulmonary capillary wedge pressure reflect the status of circulating blood volume in patient after extended transthoracic esophagectomy? J Anesth 2005;19:21–5.
14. Jones AE, Shapiro NI, Trzeciak S, et al. Lactate clearance vs. central venous oxygen saturation as goals of early sepsis therapy. JAMA 2010;303:739–46.
15. Du W, Liu D, Wang X, et al. Combining central venous-to-arterial partial pressure of carbon dioxide difference and central venous oxygen saturation to guide resuscitation in septic shock. J Crit Care 2013;28:1110.e1–5. http://dx.doi.org/ 10.1016/j.jcrc.2013.07.049.
16. Vallée F, Vallet B, Mathe O, et al. Central venous-to-arterial carbon dioxide difference: an additional target for goal-directed therapy in septic shock? Intensive Care Med 2008;34:2218–25.
17. Sakr Y, Vincent J, Schuerholz T, et al. Early- versus late-onset shock in European intensive care units. Shock 2007;28:636–43.
18. Zhen W, Schorr C, Hunter K, et al. Contrasting treatment and outcome of septic shock: presentation on hospital floors versus emergency department. Clin Med J (Engl) 2010;123:3550–3.

19. Thom O, Taylor DM, Wolfe RE, et al. Pilot study of the prevalence, outcomes and detection of occult hypoperfusion in trauma patients. Emerg Med J 2010;27: 470–2.

20. Kaplan LJ, Kellum JA. Comparison of acid-base models for prediction of hospital mortality after trauma. Shock 2008;29:662–6.

21. Jansen TC, van Bommel J, Mulder PG, et al. Prognostic value of blood lactate levels: does the clinical diagnosis at admission matter? J Trauma 2009;66: 377–85.

22. Young A, Marik PE, Sibole S, et al. Changes in end-tidal carbon dioxide and volumetric carbon dioxide as predictors of volume responsiveness in hemodynamically unstable patients. J Cardiothorac Vasc Anesth 2013;27:681–4.

23. Dunham CM, Chircihella TJ, Gruber BS, et al. In emergently ventilated trauma patients, low end-tidal CO_2 and low cardiac output are associated with hemodynamic instability, hemorrhage, abnormal pupils, and death. BMC Anesthesiology 2013;13:20. http://dx.doi.org/10.1186/1471-2253-13-20.

24. Aya HD, Cecconi M, Hamilton M, et al. Goal-directed therapy in cardiac surgery: a systematic review and meta-analysis. Br J Anaesth 2013;110:510–7.

25. Giglio MT, Marucci M, Testini M, et al. Goal-directed haemodynamic therapy and gastrointestinal complications in major surgery: a meta-analysis of randomized controlled trials. Br J Anaesth 2009;103:637–46.

26. Giglio M, Dalfino L, Puntillo F, et al. Haemodynamic goal-directed therapy in cardiac and vascular surgery. A systematic review and meta-analysis. Interact Cardiovasc Thorac Surg 2013;15:878–87.

27. Ghneim MH, Regner JL, Jupiter DC, et al. Goal directed fluid resuscitation decreases time for lactate clearance and facilitates early fascial closure in damage control surgery. Am J Surg 2013;206:995–1000.

28. Guiterrez MC, Moore PG, Liu H. Goal-directed therapy in intraoperative fluid and hemodynamic management. J Biomed Res 2013;27:357–65.

29. Haas S, Eichhorn V, Hasbach T, et al. Goal-directed fluid therapy using stroke volume variation does not result in pulmonary fluid overload in thoracic surgery requiring one-lung ventilation. Crit Care Res Pract 2012;2012:687018. http://dx.doi.org/10.1155/2012/687018.

30. Lin S, Huang C, Lin H, et al. A modified goal-directed protocol improves clinical outcomes in intensive care unit patients with septic shock: a randomized controlled trial. Shock 2006;26:551–7.

31. Forget P, Lois F, de Kock M. Goal-directed fluid management based on the pulse oximeter-derived pleth variability index reduces lactate levels and improves fluid management. Anesth Analg 2010;111:910–4.

32. Hata JS, Scotts C, Shelsky C, et al. Reduced mortality with noninvasive hemodynamic monitoring of shock. J Crit Care 2011;26:224.e1–8.

33. Benes J, Chytra I, Altmann P, et al. Intraoperative fluid optimization using stroke volume variation in high-risk surgical patients: results of prospective randomized study. Crit Care 2010;14:R118. http://dx.doi.org/10.1186/cc9070.

34. Salzwedel C, Puig J, Carstens A, et al. Perioperative goal-directed hemodynamic therapy based on radial arterial pulse pressure variation and continuous cardiac index trending reduces postoperative complications after major abdominal surgery: a multi-center, prospective, randomized study. Crit Care 2013;17: R191. Available at: http://ccforum.com/content/17/5/R191.

35. Lopes MR, Oliveira MA, Pereira VO, et al. Goal-directed fluid management based on pulse pressure variation monitoring during high-risk surgery: a pilot

randomized controlled trial. Crit Care 2007;11:R100. Available at: http://ccforum.com/content/11/5/R100.

36. Brienza N, Giglio MT, Marucci M, et al. Does perioperative hemodynamic optimization protect function in surgical patients? A meta-analytic study. Crit Care Med 2009;37:2079–90.

37. Dalfino L, Giglio MT, Puntillo F, et al. Haemodynamic goal-directed therapy and postoperative infections: earlier is better. A systematic review and meta-analysis. Crit Care 2011;15:R154. http://dx.doi.org/10.1186/cc10284.

38. Zhang J, Qiao H, He Z, et al. Intraoperative fluid management in open gastrointestinal surgery: goal-directed versus restrictive. Clinics (Sao Paulo) 2012; 67:1149–55.

39. Zheng H, Guo H, Ye J, et al. Goal-directed fluid therapy in gastrointestinal surgery in older coronary heart disease patients: randomized trial. World J Surg 2013;37:2820–9.

40. Barochia AV, Chi X, Vitberg D, et al. Bundled care for septic shock: an analysis of clinical trials. Crit Care Med 2010;38:668–78.

41. Chamberlain DJ, Willis EW, Bersten AB. The severe sepsis bundles as processes of care: a meta-analysis. Aust Crit Care 2011;24:229–43.

42. Shim HJ, Jang JY, Lee SH, et al. The effects of positive balance on the outcomes of critically ill noncardiac postsurgical patients: a retrospective cohort study. J Crit Care 2014;29:43–8.

43. Boyd JH, Forbes J, Nakada T, et al. Fluid resuscitation in septic shock: a positive fluid balance and elevated central venous pressure are associated with increased mortality. Crit Care Med 2011;39:259–65.

44. Futier E, Constantin J, Petit A, et al. Conservative vs. restrictive individualized goal-directed fluid replacement strategy in major abdominal surgery. Arch Surg 2010;145:1193–200.

45. Lobo SM, Ronchi LS, Oliveira NE, et al. Restrictive strategy of intraoperative fluid maintenance during optimization of oxygen delivery decreases major complications after high-risk surgery. Crit Care 2011;15:R226. http://dx.doi.org/10.1186/cc10466.

46. Hayes MA, Timmins AC, Yau EH, et al. Elevation of systemic oxygen delivery in the treatment of critically ill patients. N Engl J Med 1994;330:1717–22.

47. Pearse R, Dawson D, Fawcett J, et al. Early goal-directed therapy after major surgery reduces complications and duration of hospital stay. A randomised, controlled trial. Crit Care 2005;9:R687–93. Available at: http://ccforum.com/content/9/6/R687.

48. Fairchild KD, O'Shea TM. Heart rate characteristics: physiomarkers for detection of late-onset neonatal sepsis. Clin Perinatol 2010;37:581–98.

49. Godin PJ, Buchman TG. Uncoupling of biological oscillators: a complementary hypothesis concerning the pathogenesis of multiple organ dysfunction syndrome. Crit Care Med 1996;24:1107–16.

50. Pinsky MR. Complexity modeling: identify instability early. Crit Care Med 2010; 38(Suppl):S649–55.

51. Seely AJ, Christou NV. Multiple organ dysfunction syndrome: exploring the paradigm of complex nonlinear systems. Crit Care Med 2000;28:2193–200.

52. Heart rate variability: standards of measurement, physiological interpretation, and clinical use. Task Force of the European Society of Cardiology and the North American Society of Pacing and Electrophysiology. Circulation 1996;93: 1043–65.

53. Fathizadeh P, Shoemaker WC, Wo CC, et al. Autonomic activity in trauma patients based on variability of heart rate and respiratory rate. Crit Care Med 2004;32:1300–5.

54. Omboni S, Parati G, Di Rienzo M, et al. Blood pressure and heart rate in autonomic disorders: a critical review. Clin Auton Res 1996;6:171–82.

55. Kamath MV, Fallen EL. Power spectral analysis of heart rate variability: a noninvasive signature of cardiac autonomic function. Crit Rev Biomed Eng 1993;21: 245–311.

56. Kasaoka S, Nakahara T, Kawamura Y, et al. Real-time monitoring of heart rate variability in critically ill patients. J Crit Care 2010;25:313–6.

57. Kleiger RE, Miller JP, Bigger JT Jr, et al. Decreased heart rate variability and its association with increased mortality after acute myocardial infarction. Am J Cardiol 1987;59:256–62.

58. Buchan CA, Bravi A, Seely AJ. Variability analysis and the diagnosis, management, and treatment of sepsis. Curr Infect Dis Rep 2012;14:512–21.

59. Norris PR, Morris JA, Ozdas A, et al. Heart rate variability predicts trauma patient outcomes as early as 12 hours: implications for military and civilian triage. J Surg Res 2005;129:122–8.

60. Chen W, Kuo C. Characteristics of heart rate variability can predict impending shock in emergency department patients with sepsis. Acad Emerg Med 2007; 14:392–7.

61. Barnaby D, Ferrick K, Kaplan DT, et al. Heart rate variability in emergency department patients with sepsis. Acad Emerg Med 2002;9:661–70.

62. Ahmad S, Ramsay T, Huebsch L, et al. Continuous multi-parameter heart rate variability analysis heralds onset of sepsis in adults. PLoS One 2009;4:e6642. http://dx.doi.org/10.1371/journal.pone.0006642.

63. Batchinsky AI, Cooke WH, Kuusela T, et al. Loss of complexity characterizes the heart rate response to experimental hemorrhagic shock in swine. Crit Care Med 2007;35:519–25.

64. Cooke WH, Salinas J, Convertino VA, et al. Heart rate variability and its association with mortality in prehospital trauma patients. J Trauma 2006;60: 363–70.

65. Bradley B, Green GC, Batkin I, et al. Feasibility of continuous multiorgan variability analysis in the intensive care unit. J Crit Care 2012;27:218.e9–20. http://dx.doi.org/10.1016/j.jcrc.2011.09.009.

66. Cannesson M. Arterial pressure variation and goal-directed fluid therapy. J Cardiothorac Vasc Anesth 2010;24:487–97.

67. Barbeito A, Mark JB. Arterial and central venous pressure monitoring. Anesthesiol Clin 2006;24:717–35.

68. Michard F, Boussat S, Chemla D, et al. Relation between respiratory changes in arterial pulse pressure and fluid responsiveness in septic patients with acute circulatory failure. Am J Respir Crit Care Med 2000;162:134–8.

69. Huang C, Fu J, Hu H, et al. Prediction of fluid responsiveness in acute respiratory distress syndrome patients ventilated with low tidal volume and high positive end-expiratory pressure. Crit Care Med 2008;36:2810–6.

70. Zhang Z, Lu B, Sheng X, et al. Accuracy of stroke volume variation in predicting fluid responsiveness: a systematic review and meta-analysis. J Anesth 2011;25: 904–16.

71. Schereen TW, Wiesenack C, Gerlach H, et al. Goal-directed intraoperative fluid therapy guided by stroke volume and its variation in high-risk surgical patients:

a prospective randomized multicentre study. J Clin Monit Comput 2013;27: 225–33.

72. Belloni L, Pisano A, Natale A, et al. Assessment of fluid-responsiveness parameters for off-pump coronary artery bypass surgery: a comparison among LiDCO, transesophageal echocardiography, and pulmonary artery catheter. J Cardiothorac Vasc Anesth 2008;22:243–8.

73. Kramer A, Zygan D, Hawes H, et al. Pulse pressure variation predicts fluid responsiveness following coronary artery bypass surgery. Chest 2004;126: 1563–8.

74. Natalini G, Rosano A, Taranto M, et al. Arterial versus plethysmographic dynamic indices to test responsiveness for testing fluid administration in hypotensive patients: a clinical trial. Anesth Analg 2006;103:1478–84.

75. Reuter DA, Felbinger TW, Kilger E, et al. Optimizing fluid therapy in mechanically ventilated patients after cardiac surgery by on-line monitoring of left ventricular stroke volume variations. Comparison with aortic systolic pressure variations. Br J Anaesth 2002;88:124–6.

76. Tavernier B, Makhotine O, Lebuffe G, et al. Systolic pressure variation as a guide to fluid therapy in patients with sepsis-induced hypotension. Anesthesiology 1998;89:1313–21.

77. Jeleazcov C, Krajinovic L, Munster T, et al. Precision and accuracy of a new device (CNAP) for continuous non-invasive arterial pressure monitoring: assessment during general anesthesia. Br J Anaesth 2010;105:264–72.

78. Kako H, Corridore M, Rice J, et al. Accuracy of the CNAP monitor, a noninvasive continuous blood pressure device, in providing beat-to-beat blood pressure readings in pediatric patients weighing 20-40 kilograms. Paediatr Anaesth 2013;23:989–93.

79. Martina JR, Westerhof BE, van Goudoever J, et al. Noninvasive continuous arterial blood pressure monitoring with Nexfin. Anesthesiology 2012;116: 1092–103.

80. Cannesson M, Besnard C, Durand PG, et al. Relation between respiratory variations in pulse oximetry plethysmographic waveform amplitude and arterial pulse pressure in ventilated patients. Crit Care 2005;9:R562–8. Available at: http://ccforum.com/content/9/5/R562.

81. Yin JY, Ho KM. Use of plethysmographic variability index derived from the Massimo pulse oximeter to predict fluid or preload responsiveness: a systematic review and meta-analysis. Anaesthesia 2012;67:777–83.

82. O'Rourke MF. Time domain analysis of the arterial pulse in clinical medicine. Med Biol Eng Comput 2009;47:119–29.

83. Fujita Y, Hayashi D, Wada S, et al. Central venous pulse pressure analysis using an R-synchronized pressure measurement system. J Clin Monit Comput 2006; 20:385–9.

84. Roy S, Couture P, Qizilbash B, et al. Hemodynamic pressure waveform analysis in predicting volume responsiveness. J Cardiothorac Vasc Anesth 2013;27: 676–80.

85. Scheuer ML, Wilson SB. Data analysis for continuous EEG monitoring in the ICU: seeing the forest and the trees. J Clin Neurophysiol 2004;21:353–78.

86. De Melis M, Morbiducci U, Rietzschel ER, et al. Blood pressure waveform analysis by means of wavelet transform. Med Biol Eng Comput 2009;47:165–73.

87. Cohen MJ. Use of models in identification and prediction of physiology in critically ill surgical patients. Br J Surg 2012;99:487–93.

88. Dubrawski A. Detection of events in multiple streams of surveillance data: multi-variate, multi-stream and multi-dimensional approaches. In: Zeng D, Chen H, Castillo-Chavez C, et al, editors. Infectious disease informatics and bio-surveillance. New York: Springer; 2011. p. 145–71.

89. Rasouli K, Hsieh WW, Cannon AJ. Daily streamflow forecasting by machine learning methods with weather and climate inputs. J Hydrol 2012;414–415: 284–93.

90. Buckeridge DL. Outbreak detection through automated surveillance: a review of determinants of detection. J Biomed Inform 2007;40:370–9.

91. Chang Y, Yeh M, Li Y, et al. Predicting hospital-acquired infections by scoring system with simple parameters. PLoS One 2011;6:e23137. http://dx.doi.org/10.1371/journal.pone.0023137.

92. Dumont TM, Rughani AI, Tranmer BI. Prediction of symptomatic cerebral vaso-spasm after aneurysmal subarachnoid hemorrhage with an artificial neural network: feasibility and comparison with logistic regression models. World Neurosurg 2011;75:57–63.

93. Paul M, Nielsen AD, Goldberg E, et al. Prediction of specific pathogens in patients with sepsis: evaluation of TREAT, a computerized decision support system. J Antimicrob Chemother 2007;59:1204–7.

94. Purwento, Eswaran C, Logeswaran R, et al. Prediction models for early risk detection of cardiovascular event. J Med Syst 2012;36:521–31.

95. Ong ME, Ng CH, Goh K, et al. Prediction of cardiac arrest in critically ill patients presenting to the emergency department using a machine learning score incorporating heart rate variability compared with the modified early warning score. Crit Care 2012;16:R108. Available at: http://ccforum.com/content/16/3/R108.

96. Clermont G, Angus DC, DiRusso SM, et al. Predicting hospital mortality for patients in the intensive care unit: a comparison of artificial neural networks with logistic regression models. Crit Care Med 2001;29:291–6.

97. Silva A, Cortez P, Santos MF, et al. Rating organ failure via adverse events using data mining in the intensive care unit. Artif Intell Med 2008;43:179–93.

98. Ribas VJ, López JC, Ruiz-Sanmartin A, et al. Severe sepsis mortality prediction with relevance vector machines. Conf Proc IEEE Eng Med Biol Soc 2011;2011: 100–3.

99. Jaimes F, Farbiarz J, Alvarez D, et al. Comparison between logistic regression and neural networks to predict death in patients with suspected sepsis in the emergency room. Crit Care 2005;9:R150. Available at: http://ccforum.com/content/9/2/R150.

100. Gultepe E, Green JP, Nguyen H, et al. From vital signs to clinical outcomes for patients with sepsis: a machine learning basis for a clinical decision support system. J Am Med Inform Assoc 2014;21:315–25. http://dx.doi.org/10.1136/amiajnl-2013-001815.

101. Schurink CA, Lucas PJ, Hoepelman IM, et al. Computer-assisted decision support for the diagnosis and treatment of infectious diseases in intensive care units. Lancet Infect Dis 2005;5:302–12.

102. Andersson B, Andersson R, Ohlsson M, et al. Prediction of severe acute pancreatitis at admission to hospital using artificial neural networks. Pancreatology 2011;11:328–35.

103. Tang CH, Middleton PM, Savkin AV, et al. Non-invasive classification of severe sepsis and systemic inflammatory response syndrome using a nonlinear support vector machine: a preliminary study. Physiol Meas 2010; 31:775–93.

104. Xiao Y, Griffin P, Lake DE, et al. Nearest-neighbor and logistic regression analyses of clinical and heart rate characteristics in the early diagnosis of neonatal sepsis. Med Decis Making 2010;30:258–66.
105. Glass TF, Knapp J, Ambrun P, et al. Use of artificial intelligence to identify cardiovascular collapse in a model of hemorrhagic shock. Crit Care Med 2004;32: 450–6.
106. Convertino VA, Ryan KL, Rickards CA, et al. Physiological and medical monitoring for en route care of combat casualties. J Trauma 2008;64:S342–53.
107. Tarrasenko L, Hann A, Young D. Integrated monitoring and analysis for early warning of patient deterioration. Br J Anaesth 2006;97:64–8.
108. Watkinson PJ, Barber VS, Price JD, et al. A randomized controlled trial of the effect of continuous electronic physiological monitoring on the adverse event rate in high risk medical and surgical patients. Anaesthesia 2006;61: 1031–9.
109. Hravnak M, DeVita MA, Clontz A, et al. Cardiorespiratory instability before and after implementing an integrated monitoring system. Crit Care Med 2011;39: 65–72.
110. Shoemaker WC, Bayard DS, Wo CC, et al. Outcome prediction in chest injury by a mathematical search and display program. Chest 2005;128: 2739–48.
111. Shoemaker WC, Bayard DS, Botnen A, et al. Mathematical program for outcome prediction and therapeutic support for trauma beginning within 1 hr of admission: a preliminary report. Crit Care Med 2005;33:1499–506.
112. Convertino VA, Grudic G, Mulligan J, et al. Estimation of individual-specific progression to impending cardiovascular instability using arterial waveforms. J Appl Physiol (1985) 2013;115:1196–202.
113. Rothman MJ, Rothman SI, Beals J IV. Development and validation of a continuous measure of patient condition using the electronic medical record. J Biomed Inform 2013;46:837–48.
114. Bradley EH, Yakusheva O, Horwitz LI, et al. Identifying patients at risk for unplanned readmission. Med Care 2013;51:761–6.
115. Finlay GD, Rothman MJ, Smith RA. Measuring the modified early warning score and the Rothman index: advantages of utilizing the electronic medical record in an early warning system. J Hosp Med 2014;9:116–9.
116. Tepas JJ III, Rimar JM, Hsiao AL, et al. Automated analysis of electronic medical record data reflects the physiology of operative complications. Surgery 2013; 154:918–26.
117. Fairchild KD. Predictive monitoring for early detection of sepsis in neonatal ICU patients. Curr Opin Pediatr 2013;25:172–9. http://dx.doi.org/10.1097/ MOP.0b013e32835e8fe6.
118. Fairchild KD, Aschner JL. HeRO monitoring to reduce mortality in NICU patients. Res Rep Neonatol 2012;2:65–76.
119. Moorman JR, Delos JB, Flower AA, et al. Cardiovascular oscillations at the bedside: early diagnosis of neonatal sepsis using heart rate characteristics monitoring. Physiol Meas 2011;32:1821–32.
120. Griffin MP, Moorman JR. Toward the early diagnosis of neonatal sepsis and sepsis-like illness using novel heart rate analysis. Pediatrics 2001;107: 97–104.
121. Griffin MP, O'Shea TM, Bissonette EA, et al. Abnormal heart rate characteristics preceding neonatal sepsis and sepsis-like illness. Pediatr Res 2003;53: 920–6.

122. Moorman JR, Carlo WA, Kattwinkel J, et al. Mortality reduction by heart rate variability characteristic monitoring in very low birth weight neonates: a randomized controlled trial. J Pediatr 2011;159:900–6.
123. Griffin MP, Lake DE, O'Shea TM, et al. Heart rate characteristics and clinical signs in late-onset neonatal sepsis. Pediatr Res 2007;61:222–7.
124. Seely AJ, Green GC, Bravi A. Continuous multiorgan variability monitoring in critically ill patients–complexity science at the bedside. Conf Proc IEEE Eng Med Biol Soc 2011;2011:5503–6.
125. Green GC, Bradley B, Bravi A, et al. Continuous multiorgan variability analysis to track severity of organ failure in critically ill patients. J Crit Care 2013;28: 879.e1–11. http://dx.doi.org/10.1016/j.jcrc.2013.04.001.
126. Das A, Wong RC. Prediction of outcome in acute lower gastrointestinal hemorrhage: role of artificial neural network. Eur J Gastroenterol Hepatol 2007;19: 1064–9.
127. Vallée F, Fourcade O, Marty P, et al. The hemodynamic "target": a visual tool of goal-directed therapy for septic patients. Clinics (Sao Paulo) 2007;62:447–54.

Organizational Approaches to Improving Resuscitation Effectiveness

Ian J. Barbash, MD[a], Jeremy M. Kahn, MD, MS[a,b,c,*]

KEYWORDS

- Cardiac arrest • Resuscitation • Simulation • Quality improvement • Patient safety
- Hospital systems

KEY POINTS

- Improved resuscitation outcomes require not just advances in the understanding of bedside physiology but also advances in the organization of resuscitation care.
- Organizational targets for improving in-hospital resuscitation include three main domains: (1) monitoring and alerts, (2) resuscitation teams, and (3) quality improvement.
- Organizational approaches for monitoring include improved electronic health records that incorporate novel prediction models for recognizing physiologic deterioration and telemedicine for improving alert interpretation.
- Organizational approaches for resuscitation teams include formal rapid response/medical emergency teams based on managerial principals that emphasize leadership, team work, and organizational effectiveness.
- Organizational approaches for quality improvement include real-time data management strategies that feedback process and outcome data to the resuscitation team, enabling implementation of evidence-based approaches to correct specific quality deficits.
- Future research should be directed at developing novel predictive models for physiologic deterioration, improving interactions between physiology-based alarms and bedside providers, identification of the ideal components of an effective resuscitation team, and developing novel quality improvement strategies through information technology and organizational science.

Disclosures: Dr I.J. Barbash has no conflicts to disclose. Dr J.M. Kahn reports receiving in-kind research support from the Cerner Corporation, a health information technology corporation; and receiving consulting fees from the United States Department Veterans Affairs for consulting on the topic of intensive care unit telemedicine.
[a] Division of Pulmonary, Allergy, and Critical Care Medicine, University of Pittsburgh School of Medicine, 3459 Fifth Avenue, 628 Northwest, Pittsburgh, PA 15213, USA; [b] Department of Critical Care Medicine, University of Pittsburgh School of Medicine, 3550 Terrace Street, Pittsburgh, PA 15261, USA; [c] Department of Health Policy & Management, University of Pittsburgh Graduate School of Public Health, 130 De Soto Street, Pittsburgh, PA 15261, USA
* Corresponding author. Scaife Hall, Room 602-B, 3550 Terrace Street, Pittsburgh, PA 15261.
E-mail address: kahnjm@upmc.edu

Crit Care Clin 31 (2015) 165–176
http://dx.doi.org/10.1016/j.ccc.2014.08.008
0749-0704/15/$ – see front matter © 2015 Elsevier Inc. All rights reserved.

INTRODUCTION

Hemodynamic resuscitation is a central component of the care of patients with critical illness. The most common causes of critical illness world wide, including severe sepsis, trauma, acute myocardial infarction, and gastrointestinal hemorrhage, all share the common pathway of hemodynamic instability as a prelude to end organ dysfunction and death.[1] Consequently, efforts to reduce mortality and improve functional status after critical illness, regardless of cause, rest on effective resuscitation based on sound physiologic principals and evidenced-based management of shock. Indeed, many of the seminal advances in critical illness and injury in the last few decades are based on early, effective resuscitation[2,3] rather than new drugs and devices.[4]

Yet despite these advances mortality in sepsis and other forms of circulatory collapse remains depressingly high. In part, this failure is caused by the larger of failures of the health system to efficiently translate new therapies into consistent clinical care at the beside, so-called "T2" translation.[5] In severe sepsis, for example, despite strong evidence that early adequate resuscitation improves survival, only a minority of patients actually receive this therapy.[6] To address this problem, health care delivery experts are increasingly looking to the organization and management of critical care as a strategy to speed knowledge translation.[7] Under a classic model of health care quality, optimal health care structures (ie, the way health care is organized and management) are the primary determinant of the process of care, which in turn influence outcomes.[8]

Under this model, improving resuscitation outcomes requires not only a greater understand of shock physiology but also a greater understanding of the systems in which care is delivered.[9] This article describes a model for resuscitation based on modern organizational principals, describes the evidence-base for organizational approaches that might improve resuscitation outcomes, and outlines a research agenda that supports future organizational innovations in resuscitation care. Although the focus is on resuscitation in the intensive care unit (ICU), the principles described apply to resuscitation in other areas, such as the hospital ward, the emergency department, and the out-of-hospital setting.

A CONCEPTUAL MODEL FOR EFFECTIVE RESUSCITATION

Effective hospital-based resuscitation requires three primary components: (1) an afferent limb (ie, a mechanism to recognize impending physiologic deterioration), (2) an efferent limb (ie, a mechanism to delivery emergent medical care to patients with physiologic deterioration), and (3) a feedback limb (ie, a mechanism to measure and improve the quality of the afferent and efferent limbs). Each of these components has an organizational analog, depicted in **Fig. 1**. This system is similar to the neural networks by which sensory inputs are detected and elicit motor responses, which are ultimately refined by outcome-based adjustments.[10] Key principles of this model include the following: (1) in-hospital shock and death is predicated by a time period of physiologic deterioration that could be recognized by appropriate monitoring[11]: (2) rapid response teams (RRTs) and code teams can initiate treatments that improve patient outcomes, either by early response, effective resuscitation practices, or both[12]; and (3) interdisciplinary, multicomponent quality improvement based on feedback and education can improve the performance of monitoring systems and resuscitation teams.[13]

Under this model there are three domains of resuscitation effectiveness related to the organization of care: (1) monitoring and alerts (ie, the afferent limb), (2) rapid response and code teams (ie, the efferent limb), and (3) quality improvement (ie, the feedback limb) (**Table 1**). Effective resuscitation requires high-quality performance in each domain. Early warning systems and remote monitoring may help identify

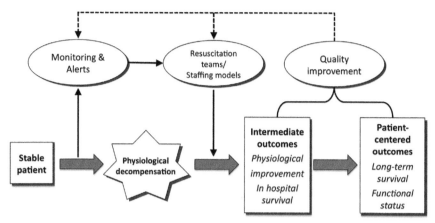

Fig. 1. Conceptual model for the organization of resuscitation care. Effective resuscitation requires three key components: (1) monitoring and identification of arrests, (2) effector teams for initiation of timely and high-quality resuscitation, and (3) feedback mechanisms for outcome measurement and improvement.

patients at risk for deterioration and prevent patients from progressing to cardiac arrest. After detection of physiologic deterioration, the resuscitation teams of the efferent limb are required to initiate timely, high-quality, evidence-based care, including administration of intravenous fluids and vasoactive agents thought to be associated with survival.[3] For patients not in the ICU, resuscitation teams need to accurately triage patients, moving those at high risk for further worsening to an ICU. Finally, feedback mechanisms must exist to accurately measure the processes and outcomes and design performance improvement interventions to refine, update, and enhance the entire system. As described in the following sections, each of these domains can be a target for improving resuscitation outcomes by improving the organization and management of care.

ORGANIZATIONAL TARGETS FOR IMPROVING RESUSCITATION EFFECTIVENESS
Monitoring and Alerts: the Afferent Limb

The first step in an effective resuscitation is the timely detection of physiologic deterioration; high-quality clinicians, either by themselves or as part of a RRT, are irrelevant

Table 1		
Organizational approaches to improving resuscitation effectiveness		
Domain	**Limb**	**Approaches**
Monitoring and alerts	Afferent	Early warning systems Integrated monitoring and decision support Telemedicine
Resuscitation teams	Efferent	Rapid response teams Physician staffing Telemedicine
Quality improvement	Feedback	Simulation training Real-time feedback Outcome measurement National quality improvement programs

if they are not alerted to patient events. Traditionally, monitoring systems were only useful in detecting cardiac arrest through telemetry.[14] However, more recently monitoring systems are used to detect deterioration well before arrest, providing time for active intervention. Thus, these systems may allow for earlier treatment and allow at-risk patients to be moved to environments in which they can be resuscitated more effectively.

Outside of the ICU, physiologic monitoring may consist of centralized cardiac telemetry, continuous pulse oximetry, and intermittent noninvasive blood pressure measurement. However, most hospitalized patients do not have these monitors in place. For example, although respiratory decompensation is an important and preventable cause of in-hospital death, only a small minority of hospital patients have respiratory monitors in place.[15] In many hospitals, standard medical and surgical wards do not have the capacity to continuously monitor patients, reserving continuous monitoring for telemetry wards that typically focus on patients at cardiac risk. Indeed, standard guidelines for the use of telemetry may overestimate risk in some patients and underestimate it in others, leading to false alarms in the former and missed arrhythmias in the latter.[16] Early detection models can help identify at-risk patients who may benefit from closer monitoring, either in situ or by a move to a higher level of care.

Although monitoring itself is not truly an organizational intervention, the act of applying prediction models to monitoring data and presenting the results of these models to providers has strong organizational underpinnings. Multiple prediction models exist, with varying inputs, weighting, and resultant differences in sensitivity and specificity for detecting deterioration (**Table 2**).[17] Several models include variations on the Early Warning Score, and others include the Medical Early Response Intervention and Therapy and the Cardiac Arrest Risk Triage. These models

Table 2
Accuracy, sensitivity, and specificity of prediction modeling for cardiac arrest

Prediction Model and Score Cutoff	IHCA Accuracy	Composite Accuracy	Sensitivity, %	Specificity, %
MEWS	0.76 (0.71–0.81)	0.75 (0.74–0.76)		
>3			67	80
>5			20	96
SEWS	0.76 (0.71–0.81)	0.76 (0.75–0.77)		
>3			55	85
>5			19	97
ViEWS	0.77 (0.72–0.82)	0.75 (0.74–0.76)		
>8			60	83
>10			29	95
CART	0.83 (0.79–0.86)	0.78 (0.77–0.79)		
>16			61	84
>24			35	95

Composite accuracy reflects receiver-operating characteristics area under the curve (95% confidence interval) for a composite measure of cardiac arrest, intensive care unit transfer, and mortality.

Abbreviations: CART, Cardiac Arrest Risk Triage; IHCA, in-hospital cardiac arrest; MEWS, Modified Early Warning System; SEWS, Standardized Early Warning System; ViEWS, VitalPAC Early Warning System.

Data from Churpek MM, Yuen TC, Edelson DP. Risk stratification of hospitalized patients on the wards. Chest 2013;143(6):1762, 1763.

incorporate various combinations of patient demographics and physiologic data to generate a risk score for predicting arrest, ICU transfer, and mortality. These models all depend on accurate collection and documentation of vital signs and, depending on the systems in place, either manual or automated calculation of risk scores followed by appropriate action on the identification of high-risk patients.

This process leaves ample room for human error. Here, the natural propensity for human error is compounded by variation in alarm signal strength and quality, false alarms, and excessive noise.[18] To overcome human error, researchers have developed "smart" monitoring systems that integrate multichannel data and alert clinicians to important trends. Smart alarms may improve the speed and accuracy with which clinicians can detect and respond to critical events.[19] Additionally, in the presence of a fully electronic medical record system, a multifaceted prediction model incorporating vital signs, laboratory values, physician orders, and patient location may prove superior to earlier models based on the detection of changes in discrete physiologic variables.[20] Early versions of such systems are under development, and initial data suggest that they may be superior to existing models for prediction and detection of physiologic deterioration.

Another organizational approach to improving monitoring and alerts is telemedicine. Telemedicine involves remote monitoring of patients using audiovisual technology. In the acute care setting, telemedicine can take several forms, including periodic consultation in the emergency department and the ICU, and continuous remote monitoring in the ICU.[21] Often, these systems include an alarm component alerting the remote monitoring personnel to physiologic deterioration. The benefit of telemedicine linked to alarms, as opposed to alarms alone, is that telemedicine reduces the opportunity costs to following up on alarms. To the degree that the alarm algorithms are imperfect, false-positives can substantially disrupt bedside work flow. Through telemedicine, remote providers can assess the accuracy of an alarm, dismiss false-positives with little effort, and react to true-positives immediately, formulating a care plan while waiting for bedside providers to reach the scene.

The conceptual rationale for telemedicine as a resuscitation tool is strong, with extensive data in other fields, such as stroke care, in which telemedicine improves the accuracy of diagnosis and timeliness of thrombolytic administration.[22] Yet, the data from ICU telemedicine are mixed, with some studies suggesting it decreased mortality and total costs, but others indicating no benefit.[23] Additionally, much of the potential benefit of telemedicine seems to derive from its role in more routine quality improvement than its role in remote monitoring.[24] Most studies emphasizing remote monitoring by itself show no impact on outcomes,[25] whereas the few studies that emphasized routine bedside quality improvement showed strong associations with outcome,[26] and there no specific data demonstrating that telemedicine improves resuscitation quality. Thus, the true role of telemedicine as an organizational adjunct to alarms and monitoring by themselves is yet to be determined.

The Efferent Limb: Resuscitation Teams

In recent decades interest emerged in team-based care for patients with trauma, myocardial infarction, and stroke, because evidence indicated that early intervention for these conditions could improve patient outcomes. Following the publication of early goal-directed treatment strategies for sepsis, it became apparent that an increasing number of hospitalized patients might benefit from intervention early in the course of clinical deterioration.[3] In the 2000s, RRTs emerged to help these patients. These teams are typically composed of physicians, nurses, and respiratory therapists, at least some of whom have training in advanced cardiovascular life support and critical care.[27] In 2005, the Institute for Healthcare Improvement included RRTs as one of six recommendations to improve health care quality.[28] The years after this recommendation saw rapid proliferation of RRTs throughout hospitals in developed countries.

Although it seems intuitive that these teams would help to improve outcomes, the data on RRTs are complex, with most available evidence showing that RRT strategy has reduced the incidence of cardiac arrest outside of the ICU without necessarily altering overall hospital mortality.[12] These studies face significant methodologic challenges. Most use a before-and-after design following implementation of a hospital-wide RRT. Before-and-after studies are notoriously difficult to interpret, because they are confounded by temporal trends and difference in case-mix between the before and after periods. Perhaps most importantly, it is difficult to reliably capture the extent to which rapid response systems contribute to early goals-of-care discussions, thereby preventing the need for resuscitation in patients who are unlikely to derive long-term benefit. At least one study demonstrated that changes in the goals of care frequently occur after RRT calls,[29] although the degree to which this occurs on a large scale is unknown. Despite these inconsistencies in the RRT literature, most hospitals in the United States continue to adopt RRTs based on their strong conceptual rationale.

Given the limitations of RRTs, a second organizational approach is education and leadership training to improve resuscitation effectiveness (ie, efforts to make response teams better, be they formal RRTs or informal resuscitation teams). Well-trained resuscitation teams can improve resuscitation outcomes by facilitating aggressive fluid resuscitation and other evidence-based treatments. Here, several lessons can be drawn from the literature on in-hospital cardiac arrest, in which two of the most important predictors of mortality are delayed defibrillation and interruption of chest compressions.[30] Compared with ad hoc teams, those with prespecified leadership and organized roles perform earlier defibrillation and maintain greater "hands-on time" during simulated arrests.[31] Other simulation studies indicate that initial resuscitation by nonphysician first responders may delay defibrillation in arrest.[32] Other important factors may include effective communication or well-defined roles.[33] These findings are supported by observations from in situ surprise simulations of cardiac arrest on hospital wards, which demonstrate improved quality of cardiopulmonary resuscitation after arrival of a code team compared with the resuscitation efforts of the first responder hospital staff.[34] The major conclusion from these studies is that it is not enough for resuscitation teams to simply exist and respond to cardiac arrest; rather, they must function with good leadership and effective communication.[35,36]

The strong conceptual model for an impact of high-functioning teams on the quality of resuscitation efforts begs the question of why this beneficial effect has been difficult to demonstrate or detect in clinical practice. First, there is a difference between resuscitation from cardiac arrest and triage or treatment of a deteriorating patient, which is the more typical situation encountered by a RRT. Cardiac arrest care is highly protocolized and algorithm-based, whereas nonarrest resuscitation requires intellectual nuance that resists protocolization. Another possible explanation often suggested in the RRT literature is that the monitoring systems in place during the studies may not identify those patients who would most benefit from care from an RRT. As a result, RRTs may be called on the wrong patients, or may be called too late to have an impact. Thus, an important strategy may be to reduce the "cultural" barriers to calling an RRT; if bedside nurses are uncomfortable calling for help or afraid of repercussions from unnecessary calls, an opportunity for early intervention may be missed.[37]

Another important aspect of the resuscitation team is the leader, who should have appropriate time, training, and expertise to manage a complex resuscitation.

Substantial data suggest that the presence of a trained intensivist physician is associated with improved outcomes in the ICU.[38] Although the exact mechanism of intensivist physician staffing is unknown, it may in part be caused by improved resuscitation at the bedside.[39] For example, adding intensivist physicians to the ICU increased the chance of receiving a sepsis resuscitation bundle, although these effects were not statistically significant.[40]

Here, telemedicine may also play a role. A resuscitation team might have all the necessary components to deliver high-quality care, but lack an effective leader for coordination and key decision making. Telemedicine could be used to remotely bring an experienced leader to the team. This approach would be analogous to stroke telemedicine, in which expertise required but not readily available at all hospitals is delivered remotely as needed rather than all the time.[22] If the technology required could be deployed rapidly, team leaders could review data, coordinate care, and make key decisions from a remote location, expanding access to this essential component of hospital-based critical care.

The Feedback Limb: Quality Improvement

The third major organizational approach to improving resuscitation outcomes is quality improvement. Broadly defined, quality improvement is a systematic, data-driven approach to improving health care processes and outcomes. Quality improvement in resuscitation systems requires multiple components: data to measure quality through the process of care (ie, timely arrival and treatment) and outcomes of care (ie, postresuscitation survival and functional status); feedback mechanisms to present that data on processes and outcomes back to providers in ways that are meaningful and actionable; and organizational-based approaches to improve quality based on a critical interpretation of the data.

The first step is obtaining data—that which cannot be measured cannot be improved. Without reliable outcome data it is impossible to know whether interventions are having their intended effect. Therefore, all hospitals should ideally maintain accurate and up-to-date databases of clinical outcomes. Hospitals with RRTs should maintain data on the frequency of calls, the reasons for the calls, the actions of the team, and the subsequent outcomes of the patients. These databases are important for not only broadly measuring resuscitation effectiveness but also identifying targets for quality improvement, the so-called "needs assessment" part of the quality improvement process.[13] For example, one hospital seeking to improve outcomes might find that the RRT teams are not consistently called before arrest, whereas another hospital might find that fluids are not administered in a timely fashion. These different findings would lead to different interventions.

In addition to such hospital-wide databases, technologies exist that can provide real-time quality to resuscitation teams. In cardiac arrest, investigational devices can be used to monitor the effectiveness of chest compressions and ventilation in simulated and actual hospital code environments.[41] These devices provide immediate feedback to providers, allowing them to improve the quality of their resuscitation efforts. This technology is still experimental, and has not yet shown an improvement in return of spontaneous circulation or survival to hospital discharge. However, early data suggest that real-time quality monitoring is an important frontier for improving resuscitation effectiveness.

Another source of data on resuscitation effectiveness is through surveys of providers. Most simply take the form of semistructured interviews designed to elicit opportunities for improvement from the perspectives of front-line practitioners. More advanced approaches involve the used of validated scoring systems for team effectiveness. Two scoring systems currently exist: team emergency assessment measure and observational skill-based clinical assessment tool for resuscitation.[42,43] They are designed to assess teamwork and nontechnical skills during resuscitation, have good interrater reliability, and can distinguish higher- from lower-performing teams in simulation studies. These tools may help assess which interventions improve the performance of resuscitation teams in the simulation laboratory, and thereby to develop strategies that might improve outcomes when deployed in the clinical arena.

After quality deficiencies have been identified, it is then necessary to design interventions to target them, with a goal of improving the processes and outcomes of care. Many of these approaches are straightforward, such as simulation training in basic life support and advanced life support.[41] Others are more difficult, such as targeting a culture change to make it easier for ward nurses to call RRTs to the bedside, or leadership training to improve overall resuscitation team functioning. Yet early data suggest that these interventions, particularly when multimodal involving education and feedback, can be remarkably effective. For example, the Surviving Sepsis Campaign, a large-scale quality improvement initiative designed in part around early sepsis resuscitation, has been associated with substantial improvements in sepsis survival in Spain and in the United States.[44,45]

The Surviving Sepsis Campaign is focused on specific care processes, such as the use of physiologic parameters to drive resuscitation. Perhaps more challenging is whether quality improvement efforts can address team function, leadership, and communication. Leadership "targets" do exist based on observations of resuscitation teams. Leaders who play a coordinating role, assign roles, communicate openly and clearly, and avoid direct hands-on involvement in the resuscitation are more likely help their teams achieve resuscitation goals. Based on these and other studies, Hunziker and colleagues[35] have outlined a framework for leadership during resuscitation (**Box 1**).

Box 1
Principles for demonstrating and teaching effective leadership

Effective leadership principles

  Evaluate existing leadership before interjecting with new leadership

  Identify progress aloud and elicit contributions

  Identify problems by asking questions that highlight them

  As a team leader, avoid direct, hands-on involvement; assign tasks

  Facilitate open and effective communication (affirmative statements, closed-loop communication)

Effective leadership teaching

  Explain the importance and impact of leadership

  Demonstrate difference in leadership styles

  Monitor adherence to leadership principles and algorithms; provide feedback

  Facilitate open and effective communication

  Speak clearly and concisely

Adapted from Hunziker S, Johansson AC, Tschan F, et al. Teamwork and leadership in cardiopulmonary resuscitation. J Am Coll Cardiol 2011;57(24):2381–8. http://dx.doi.org/10.1016/j.jacc.2011.03.017; with permission.

FUTURE DIRECTIONS AND AREAS FOR RESEARCH

The conceptual model outlined in this article (that of a sensorimotor loop requiring sensing, action, and feedback) provides a framework for a systems-based approach to improving resuscitation outcomes. The existing literature lends support to this model and its components, providing some concrete targets for organizational approaches to improve resuscitation effectiveness. However, many questions remain and should be the focus of future research.

Monitoring and Alerts

- Can useful, real-time, validated prediction models be developed that incorporate multichannel input from the electronic medical record to improve sensitivity and specificity over existing models?
- Will implementation of new and existing prediction rules lead to new care processes resulting in improved clinical outcomes, or merely strengthen existing processes leading to static outcomes?
- How can alerts for potential physiologic deterioration be made "smarter," both by improving sensitivity and specificity; and by improving the user interface allowing for more effective human-alarm interactions and reducing alarm fatigue?
- How can early identification of at-risk patients facilitate code status discussions and help to prevent unwanted or inappropriate resuscitation?
- What is the best way of integrating telemedicine into monitoring?

Resuscitation Teams

- What is the ideal composition and leadership of a resuscitation team?
- Should resuscitation teams be static, comprised of the same individuals over and over again, or dynamic, comprised of different providers at different times?
- Should resuscitation teams be dedicated to resuscitation or should they be allowed to have other clinical duties, such as working in the ICU?
- Are different leadership styles more suitable to different clinical situations (ie, cardiac arrest vs ICU rounds)?
- What is the best way of integrating telemedicine into resuscitation?

Feedback and Quality Improvement

- Can existing and newly developed audiovisual biofeedback technology be consistently integrated into resuscitation efforts?
- Will these feedback mechanisms improve resuscitation outcomes?
- Can we develop metrics to assess not only a team as a whole, but also the style and quality of its leadership?
- Does simulation-based team training reliably translate into improved patient-centered outcomes after resuscitation?

SUMMARY

Although it is tempting to seek improvement in patient outcomes via new, and often expensive, medical technologies, simple systems-based interventions frequently yield equal if not greater changes. For decades, critical care research focused on understanding and altering the physiology of sepsis, investing millions of dollars in trials of various investigational agents. In the end, early and appropriate antibiotics, early restoration of the circulation, prevention of ICU complications, and the systems needed to address the failure to achieve those goals proved the most important aspects of improving outcomes for patients with septic shock. Thus, although the last decade has seen a rapid expansion in the understanding of resuscitation physiology, we must not lose sight of the systems necessary to complement innovations in resuscitation science and improve patient outcomes. This effort requires systems that identify patients at risk, resuscitation teams with effective leaders who can rapidly implement high-quality evidenced-based, and feedback mechanisms that identify changes in patient outcome and facilitate quality improvement in resuscitation systems.

REFERENCES

1. Carrico CJ, Meakins JL, Marshall JC, et al. Multiple-organ-failure syndrome. Arch Surg 1986;121(2):196–208.
2. MacKenzie EJ, Rivara FP, Jurkovich GJ, et al. A national evaluation of the effect of trauma-center care on mortality. N Engl J Med 2006;354(4):366–78. http://dx.doi.org/10.1056/NEJMsa052049.
3. Rivers E, Nguyen B, Havstad S, et al. Early goal-directed therapy in the treatment of severe sepsis and septic shock. N Engl J Med 2001;345(19):1368–77. http://dx.doi.org/10.1056/NEJMoa010307.
4. Ranieri VM, Thompson BT, Barie PS, et al. Drotrecogin alfa (activated) in adults with septic shock. N Engl J Med 2012;366(22):2055–64. http://dx.doi.org/10.1056/NEJMoa1202290.
5. Sinuff T, Muscedere J, Adhikari NK, et al. Knowledge translation interventions for critically ill patients. Crit Care Med 2013;41(11):2627–40. http://dx.doi.org/10.1097/CCM.0b013e3182982b03.
6. Mikkelsen ME, Gaieski DF, Goyal M, et al. Factors associated with nonadherence to early goal-directed therapy in the ED. Chest 2010;138(3):551–8. http://dx.doi.org/10.1378/chest.09-2210.
7. Carmel S, Rowan K. Variation in intensive care unit outcomes: a search for the evidence on organizational factors. Curr Opin Crit Care 2001;7(4):284–96.
8. Donabedian A. The quality of medical care. Science 1978;200(4344):856–64.
9. Kahn JM, Rubenfeld GD. Translating evidence into practice in the intensive care unit: the need for a systems-based approach. J Crit Care 2005;20(3):204–6. http://dx.doi.org/10.1016/j.jcrc.2005.06.001.
10. Stephenson-Jones M, Kardamakis AA, Robertson B, et al. Independent circuits in the basal ganglia for the evaluation and selection of actions. Proc Natl Acad Sci U S A 2013;110(38):E3670–9. http://dx.doi.org/10.1073/pnas.1314815110.
11. Schein RM, Hazday N, Pena M, et al. Clinical antecedents to in-hospital cardiopulmonary arrest. Chest 1990;98(6):1388–92.
12. Chan PS, Jain R, Nallmothu BK, et al. Rapid response teams: a systematic review and meta-analysis. Arch Intern Med 2010;170(1):18–26. http://dx.doi.org/10.1001/archinternmed.2009.424.
13. Curtis JR, Cook DJ, Wall RJ, et al. Intensive care unit quality improvement: a "how-to" guide for the interdisciplinary team. Crit Care Med 2006;34(1):211–8.
14. Drew BJ, Califf RM, Funk M, et al. Practice standards for electrocardiographic monitoring in hospital settings: an American Heart Association scientific statement from the Councils on Cardiovascular Nursing, Clinical Cardiology, and Cardiovascular Disease in the Young: endorsed by the International Society of Computerized Electrocardiology and the American Association of Critical-Care Nurses. Circulation 2004;110(17):2721–46. http://dx.doi.org/10.1161/01.CIR.0000145144.56673.59.

15. Chon GR, Lee J, Shin Y, et al. Clinical outcomes of witnessed and monitored cases of in-hospital cardiac arrest in the general ward of a university hospital in Korea. Respir Care 2013;58(11):1937–44. http://dx.doi.org/10.4187/respcare.02448.

16. Estrada CA, Rosman HS, Prasad NK, et al. Evaluation of guidelines for the use of telemetry in the non-intensive-care setting. J Gen Intern Med 2000;15(1):51–5.

17. Churpek MM, Yuen TC, Edelson DP. Risk stratification of hospitalized patients on the wards. Chest 2013;143(6):1758–65. http://dx.doi.org/10.1378/chest.12-1605.

18. Edworthy J, Hellier E. Alarms and human behaviour: implications for medical alarms. Br J Anaesth 2006;97(1):12–7. http://dx.doi.org/10.1093/bja/ael114.

19. Görges M, Winton P, Koval V, et al. An evaluation of an expert system for detecting critical events during anesthesia in a human patient simulator: a prospective randomized controlled study. Anesth Analg 2013;117(2):380–91. http://dx.doi.org/10.1213/ANE.0b013e3182975b63.

20. Churpek MM, Yuen TC, Park SY, et al. Using electronic health record data to develop and validate a prediction model for adverse outcomes in the wards. Crit Care Med 2014;42:841–8. http://dx.doi.org/10.1097/CCM.0000000000000038.

21. Kahn JM, Hill NS, Lilly CM, et al. The research agenda in ICU telemedicine: a statement from the Critical Care Societies Collaborative. Chest 2011;140(1):230–8. http://dx.doi.org/10.1378/chest.11-0610.

22. Schwamm LH, Holloway RG, Amarenco P, et al. A review of the evidence for the use of telemedicine within stroke systems of care: a scientific statement from the American Heart Association/American Stroke Association. Stroke 2009;40(7):2616–34. http://dx.doi.org/10.1161/STROKEAHA.109.192360.

23. Wilcox ME, Adhikari NK. The effect of telemedicine in critically ill patients: systematic review and meta-analysis. Crit Care 2012;16(4):R127. http://dx.doi.org/10.1186/cc11429.

24. Kahn JM. The use and misuse of ICU telemedicine. JAMA 2011;305(21):2227–8. http://dx.doi.org/10.1001/jama.2011.716.

25. Thomas EJ, Lucke JF, Wueste L, et al. Association of telemedicine for remote monitoring of intensive care patients with mortality, complications, and length of stay. JAMA 2009;302(24):2671–8. http://dx.doi.org/10.1001/jama.2009.1902.

26. Lilly CM, Cody S, Zhao H, et al. Hospital mortality, length of stay, and preventable complications among critically ill patients before and after tele-ICU reengineering of critical care processes. JAMA 2011;305(21):2175–83. http://dx.doi.org/10.1001/jama.2011.697.

27. Hillman K, Parr M, Flabouris A, et al. Redefining in-hospital resuscitation: the concept of the medical emergency team. Resuscitation 2001;48(2):105–10.

28. Gosfield AG, Reinertsen JL. The 100,000 lives campaign: crystallizing standards of care for hospitals. Health Aff (Millwood) 2005;24(6):1560–70. http://dx.doi.org/10.1377/hlthaff.24.6.1560.

29. Stelfox HT, Hemmelgarn BR, Bagshaw SM, et al. Intensive care unit bed availability and outcomes for hospitalized patients with sudden clinical deterioration. Arch Intern Med 2012;172(6):467–74. http://dx.doi.org/10.1001/archinternmed.2011.2315.

30. Chan PS, Krumholz HM, Nichol G, et al. American Heart Association National Registry of Cardiopulmonary Resuscitation Investigators. Delayed time to defibrillation after in-hospital cardiac arrest. N Engl J Med 2008;358(1):9–17. http://dx.doi.org/10.1056/NEJMoa0706467.

31. Hunziker S, Tschan F, Semmer NK, et al. Hands-on time during cardiopulmonary resuscitation is affected by the process of teambuilding: a prospective

randomised simulator-based trial. BMC Emerg Med 2009;9:3. http://dx.doi.org/10.1186/1471-227X-9-3.

32. Marsch SC, Tschan F, Semmer N, et al. Performance of first responders in simulated cardiac arrests. Crit Care Med 2005;33(5):963–7.

33. Marsch SC, Müller C, Marquardt K, et al. Human factors affect the quality of cardiopulmonary resuscitation in simulated cardiac arrests. Resuscitation 2004; 60(1):51–6. http://dx.doi.org/10.1016/j.resuscitation.2003.08.004.

34. Mondrup F, Brabrand M, Folkestad L, et al. In-hospital resuscitation evaluated by in situ simulation: a prospective simulation study. Scand J Trauma Resusc Emerg Med 2011;19:55. http://dx.doi.org/10.1186/1757-7241-19-55.

35. Hunziker S, Johansson AC, Tschan F, et al. Teamwork and leadership in cardiopulmonary resuscitation. J Am Coll Cardiol 2011;57(24):2381–8. http://dx.doi.org/10.1016/j.jacc.2011.03.017.

36. Fernandez Castelao E, Russo SG, Riethmüller M, et al. Effects of team coordination during cardiopulmonary resuscitation: a systematic review of the literature. J Crit Care 2013;28(4):504–21. http://dx.doi.org/10.1016/j.jcrc.2013.01.005.

37. Bagshaw SM, Mondor EE, Scouten C, et al. A survey of nurses' beliefs about the medical emergency team system in a Canadian tertiary hospital. Am J Crit Care 2010;19(1):74–83. http://dx.doi.org/10.4037/ajcc2009532.

38. Pronovost PJ, Angus DC, Dorman T, et al. Physician staffing patterns and clinical outcomes in critically ill patients: a systematic review. JAMA 2002;288(17): 2151–62.

39. Kahn JM, Brake H, Steinberg KP. Intensivist physician staffing and the process of care in academic medical centres. Qual Saf Health Care 2007;16(5):329–33. http://dx.doi.org/10.1136/qshc.2007.022376.

40. Gajic O, Afessa B, Hanson AC, et al. Effect of 24-hour mandatory versus on-demand critical care specialist presence on quality of care and family and provider satisfaction in the intensive care unit of a teaching hospital. Crit Care Med 2008;36(1):36–44. http://dx.doi.org/10.1097/01.CCM.0000297887.84347.85.

41. Abella BS, Edelson DP, Kim S, et al. CPR quality improvement during in-hospital cardiac arrest using a real-time audiovisual feedback system. Resuscitation 2007;73(1):54–61. http://dx.doi.org/10.1016/j.resuscitation.2006.10.027.

42. Cooper S, Cant R, Porter J, et al. Rating medical emergency teamwork performance: development of the Team Emergency Assessment Measure (TEAM). Resuscitation 2010;81(4):446–52. http://dx.doi.org/10.1016/j.resuscitation.2009.11.027.

43. Walker S, Brett S, McKay A, et al. Observational skill-based clinical assessment tool for resuscitation (OSCAR): development and validation. Resuscitation 2011; 82(7):835–44. http://dx.doi.org/10.1016/j.resuscitation.2011.03.009.

44. Levy MM, Dellinger RP, Townsend SR, et al. The Surviving Sepsis Campaign: results of an international guideline-based performance improvement program targeting severe sepsis. Crit Care Med 2010;38(2):367–74. http://dx.doi.org/10.1097/CCM.0b013e3181cb0cdc.

45. Ferrer R, Artigas A, Levy MM, et al. Improvement in process of care and outcome after a multicenter severe sepsis educational program in Spain. JAMA 2008; 299(19):2294–303. http://dx.doi.org/10.1001/jama.299.19.2294.

Index

Note: Page numbers of article titles are in **boldface** type.

Crit Care Clin 31 (2015) 177–186
http://dx.doi.org/10.1016/S0749-0704(14)00092-X
0749-0704/15/$ – see front matter © 2015 Elsevier Inc. All rights reserved.

criticalcare.theclinics.com

Moving?

Make sure your subscription moves with you!

To notify us of your new address, find your **Clinics Account Number** (located on your mailing label above your name), and contact customer service at:

Email: journalscustomerservice-usa@elsevier.com

800-654-2452 (subscribers in the U.S. & Canada)
314-447-8871 (subscribers outside of the U.S. & Canada)

Fax number: 314-447-8029

Elsevier Health Sciences Division
Subscription Customer Service
3251 Riverport Lane
Maryland Heights, MO 63043

*To ensure uninterrupted delivery of your subscription, please notify us at least 4 weeks in advance of move.

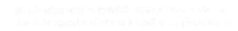